LIFE AND LOVE

Towards a Christian dialogue on
bioethical questions

By the same author
DIVORCE AND SECOND MARRIAGE

LIFE AND LOVE

Towards a Christian dialogue on bioethical questions

Kevin T. Kelly

COLLINS

Collins Liturgical Publications
8 Grafton Street, London W1X 3LA

Distributed in USA by
Harper & Row, Publishers, Inc., San Francisco
Icehouse One — 401
151 Union Street, San Francisco, CA 94111-1299

Distributed in Canada by
Novalis, Box 9700, Terminal,
375 Rideau St, Ottawa, Ontario K1G 4B4

Distributed in Ireland by
Educational Company of Ireland
21 Talbot Street, Dublin 1

Collins Liturgical Australia
PO Box 316, Blackburn, Victoria 3130

Collins Liturgical New Zealand
PO Box 1, Auckland

ISBN 0 00 599968 5
© 1987 Kevin Kelly
First published 1987

Typesetting by John Swain and Sons (Glasgow) Limited
Printed in Great Britain by Richard Clay Ltd, Bungay, Suffolk

Contents

Introduction

Most people can remember exactly where they were when certain events of key historical significance took place. I remember that I was helping out in a parish on the outskirts of New York in Summer 1978 when the news broke about the birth of Louise Brown. She entered the history books as the first baby to be born who had been conceived in a laboratory in a glass dish (*in vitro*). Her birth made head-lines in all the major newspapers throughout the world. Louise Brown was not simply another 'first', another name to go into the record books. Her birth signalled a break-through for medical science and technology which may be even more far-reaching in its implications than humankind's first step on the moon. Human agency had stepped in and exercised control in a process which throughout history had always tended to be regarded as the work of God's providence.

Reactions to Louise's birth were mixed. Most people could feel in tune with her parents' great joy at being able to have a child of their own. People could also appreciate that her birth represented an extraordinary achievement of modern medical science and technology. Dr Edwards and Mr Steptoe became world-famous overnight. Yet a note of caution was also voiced by many commentators. The birth of Louise Brown was seen to have a significance far beyond that of providing a remedy for the infertility of some couples. It also opened up the possibility of radically changing the natural processes of human reproduction which had been in operation since the beginning of human history. Even prior to the birth of Louise Brown the moral and ethical questions linked to this possibility were already being explored by some writers in the field of Christian ethics. However, until Louise was born, this was viewed as purely speculative writing about a future that might never happen. The birth of Louise changed all that. In-vitro fertilisation and reproductive medicine came into their own as major issues in the field of medical ethics. Since 1978 the literature on this topic has been increasing and multiplying.

The debate was not restricted to professionals in the field of medical ethics. Understandably enough these issues captured the public imagination. The far-reaching implications of reproductive medicine soon began to dawn on people at large. As a result, in July 1982 Her Majesty's Government established a Committee of Enquiry into Human Fertilisation and

Embryology chaired by Dame Mary Warnock. Its terms of reference were:

> 'To consider recent and potential developments in medicine and science related
> to human fertilisation and embryology; to consider what policies and safe-
> guards should be applied, including consideration of the social, ethical and
> legal implications of these developments; and to make recommendations.'

Among the submissions sent in to the Committee were nearly fifty from
the different churches and church organisations in the United Kingdom.
Furthermore, when the Committee's report was finally published in July
1984 many of the churches produced official responses to its findings.

Public interest and concern has not waned since the publication of the
Warnock Report. Both the press and television have kept the issue before
people's minds. Moreover, although the Warnock Report was widely welcomed as a serious attempt to grapple with the complex ethical, legal and
social problems involved in advances in reproductive medicine, it has not
generally been viewed as the final word on the issue. Its standing is more
that of a very valuable and authoritative position paper which has provided an excellent starting point for responsible debate within the community.

The fact that nearly fifty churches or church organisations sent in submissions to the Warnock Committee shows that Christians view the issue
with some concern. The churches obviously believe that they have something of value to contribute to the discussion.

Are the churches all saying the same thing on this issue? Did the fifty or
so church submissions to the Warnock Committee speak with a common
voice or were the Committee confronted with a multiplicity of different
positions all claiming to be Christian?

These are important questions since the debate is far from over. Until
now the Government has not shown any strong political will to introduce
legislation on this important topic. Whether the DHSS consultation paper,
Legislation on Human Infertility Services and Embryo Research, issued in
December 1986 is an indication that the Government is at long last slowly
beginning to move is unclear. It is expressly intended to initiate a further
period of consultation: 'The Government has indicated on a number of
occasions its intention to introduce comprehensive legislation. However,
the range and complexity of the issues raised by the Warnock Report and
the strength and diversity of opinion expressed make it desirable that there
should be a further period for consultation before any legislation is
drafted.' (p.4) There is no doubt that eventually there will be some legisla-

tion on this matter. In a democratic society and on a non-party issue such as this, what form this legislation will take will be determined largely by public opinion.

The Christian churches would not claim that it is their role to dictate to the general public what they should think on such an issue. However, they would claim that it is their responsibility to make sure that the public debate does not lack that essential ingredient which is provided by the Christian vision of the meaning of human life. This vision focuses particularly on the dignity of the human person and of the human family's responsibility for all its members (both living and yet to be born) and for the whole of God's creation.

It is understandable that the different Christian churches will speak in their own distinctive accents when they contribute to the debate. Each church will introduce its own particular flavour, as it were; each will approach the issue from the perspective of its own special tradition. That kind of variety can add a certain richness and breadth of vision to the Christian contribution. However, an accent must not distort the basic message; a flavour must not take away the taste of the principal ingredient; and a perspective must not allow the main object of vision to drop out of sight.

If the Christian churches differ in their contributions to the debate, one would not expect these differences to be over essentials. At best their differences should be complementary perspectives, each enriching the vision still further; at worst their differences should be no more than disagreements about non-essentials. If the differences between the churches go deeper than that and are tantamount to contradictory positions on fundamental issues, the voice of Christian witness becomes a broken and discordant sound. Far from enriching the debate with the Christian contribution, it will have the very opposite effect and will ensure that any Christian contribution that is made will be lost in all the confusion created by conflicting church voices.

To avoid the tragedy of such a counter-witness it is essential that the Christian churches listen to what each other is saying on this issue. Interchurch dialogue would seem to be a pre-requisite for this. Moreover, it should be an inter-church dialogue which takes place not just behind the closed doors of committee rooms but at the more general level of public discussion between ordinary members of the different churches. If the Christian view-point is to have any effect on public opinion, it must itself be the opinion of the vast numbers of ordinary Christians who comprise a major sector of the public in Great Britain. That will hardly be the case if serious Christian discussion of these issues is made the sacred preserve of those involved at a professional level in Christian ethics. If the different churches are to contribute a basic shared Christian vision to the debate, it needs to be a vision which is shared first of all by their own members.

It is against that general background that this book is written both as a reaction and as a contribution.

It is a reaction to the fact that at present inter-church dialogue seems to be concerned almost exclusively with doctrinal matters. It is not reacting against the urgent need to discuss such doctrinal matters. What it is reacting against is the fact that the need to discuss ethical issues seems to be completely overlooked. For some people this is a sign that the churches regard ethical issues as of secondary importance; for others, it shows that the churches are wary of putting ethical issues on the agenda for inter-church dialogue lest they prove to be too divisive. For my own part, I firmly believe that there is an urgent need for serious ecumenical dialogue on a whole variety of issues concerned with both personal and social ethics. The main reason for such dialogue is so that the Christian churches can be more effective in bringing the vision of the Gospel to bear on the burning issues facing society today. However, another important reason is that the ethical differences between the churches could well prove to be a time-bomb which, unless defused in time, might eventually explode in our faces and destroy the progress towards unity which is being made through doctrinal dialogue. I feel sure that this is particularly true of any moves towards unity which involve the Roman Catholic church.

As well as being written as a reaction to this lack of dialogue, this book is also meant to be a modest contribution which might help to clear the ground to make such inter-church dialogue possible on some of the complex ethical issues raised by modern advances in reproductive medicine.

In line with this purpose, I have tried to examine and compare the various 'official' or quasi-official statements of the main-line churches in Britain on these issues. This methodology carries its own in-built weakness since the different church positions on authority mean that in comparing such 'official' statements I am not comparing like to like. A statement approved by the Methodist Conference, for instance, is a very different kind of authoritative utterance from a declaration issued by a Vatican Congregation or a report from the Church of England Board for Social Responsibility. Nevertheless, despite that difficulty I have felt that there is some usefulness in this method. In its own way each church is trying to articulate how it discerns the right way forward in these difficult and perplexing issues which will affect both present and future generations. At that level each church, depending on how it understands its teaching mission as church, is attempting to speak with as much authority as it sees to be available to it.

How far the 'official' teaching of any particular church is shared by its members is a very important issue but one which I have neither time nor space to investigate. Clearly some churches have a much stronger interpretation of their teaching authority than others. However, even within a church like the Roman Catholic church, which has probably the strongest interpretation of teaching authority, there can at times be found strong disagreement with 'official' teaching, especially in the area of personal and sexual morality. The possibility of such dissent from non-infallible teaching has long been regarded as acceptable by theologians but it has usually been restricted to the private or professional sphere. Whether such dissent should still be limited to the private and professional sphere is a question which is being vigorously debated in the Roman Catholic church at present. The way the church exercises its teaching mission has to take account of the new age in which we are living; the communications explosion has resulted in widespread public interest in theological and moral issues and adult Christian education has become a high pastoral priority in the church. Certainly, for the purposes of this book the mere fact that certain moral positions are stated authoritatively in official Roman Catholic teaching documents should not be taken as necessarily implying that such positions are the only ones represented in Roman Catholic theological thinking.

This point needs to be made at this early stage in the book. It will obviate any need to use the expression 'official Roman Catholic teaching'. The constant repetition of such a phrase could be interpreted in a pejorative sense and could give the impression that there is normally a deep divide between 'official Roman Catholic teaching' and what is believed by many Roman Catholics. That is not true. Nevertheless, it cannot be denied that disagreements do exist and some of them touch on issues related to the theme of this book.

Obviously, in those Christian churches which interpret their teaching authority less strongly, it is only to be expected that their 'official' teaching, especially on specific matters relating to the moral field, will on occasion be questioned by some of their theologians or ordinary church members.

My aim in this book is to undertake three distinct, though closely related, tasks:- (1) to discern any points of common agreement or possible convergence between the churches; (2) to pin-point the major differences between the churches on these issues and to explore why such disagreements exist; (3) to look at the possibilities for dialogue between the churches on the issues under consideration.

As my work progressed, it became even clearer that there was in fact a fair measure of disagreement among the churches and at times this disagreement was quite substantial in its practical implications. Where such disagreement occurred, it was frequently the Roman Catholic church which was the odd one out. Moreover, the major items of disagreement seemed to be closely related to the positions adopted by the churches on two other moral issues of practical importance. One was the issue of artificial contraception; this was because that issue raised the question of how far it is morally acceptable to separate the relational and procreational aspects of marriage. The other was the issue of abortion; that was because abortion high-lighted the question: is the same reverence owed to the embryo as to every other living human being? At one stage in planning the book I considered treating contraception, abortion and in-vitro fertilisation as three separate topics. However, in the end I decided that the only way to keep things within manageable proportions was to keep in-vitro fertilisation as the main point of focus. Nevertheless, it was clear that the position of the different churches on abortion needed a chapter of its own since it was in discussing abortion that the various churches had worked out their respective positions on the status of the embryo which they then applied to the issue of IVF and the experimental research linked to it. However, the separation of the relational and procreational aspects of marriage did not seem to demand such a detailed treatment in a separate chapter. It seemed feasible to work that into the section on IVF itself.

While this book was in the final stages of preparation, the ordination of women was a burning topic, especially within the Church of England. Most people would probably agree that the point at issue here is not simply whether women can be ordained priests. It also concerns the full participation of women in decision-making at all levels of church life. When I decided to concentrate on the 'official' or quasi-official statements of the different Christian churches, I was fully aware that this would effectively exclude from the discussion any contribution from a woman's perspective. Consequently, from the earliest planning stage I was determined to try to remedy this serious deficiency in some way or other. That explains the inclusion of Chapter 5 which tries to listen to what some women are saying about IVF and the issues related to it. A further reason for including such a chapter is that the issues related to reproductive medicine are of particular concern to women since they are affected most directly by them. It is crucial that their voice be heard loud and clear. I have tried as far as possible to make it a 'listening' chapter. This explains the extensive use of quotations in that chapter and the resulting predominance of feminist literature in the bibliography. I have shown the preliminary version of this chapter to a number of women, all of them strong feminists in their different ways. I am grateful to them for their encouragement and for their criticisms.

The primary purpose of this book is to argue the case for ecumenical dialogue in the field of Christian ethics. I have chosen in-vitro fertilisation as a burning contemporary issue which highlights the need for such ecumenical dialogue. Moreover, it has the added advantage that it provides a 'new' context for re-examining the two 'old' issues of contraception and abortion which have created a deep division between some churches and also among individual Christians.

Since the book's main focus is ecumenical, it is very appropriate that it should have been written at The Queen's College, Birmingham, the only ecumenical Theological College in Britain. My year's residence there was made possible through the ecumenical generosity of both the College Council who very kindly selected me to be Research Fellow for 1985-86 and the Fellowship Trustees who are responsible for the funding of the Fellowship. I am deeply grateful to both these bodies. But for them I would never have been able to write this book. I am also grateful to the Reverend Gordon Wakefield, the Principal of The Queen's College, who not only acted as my tutor but who inspired me deeply by his profound ecumenical commitment and spirituality. I would like to thank all the Staff and Students of the College who made me feel so welcome in their midst, with a special word of thanks going to Sheila Russell, the Librarian, and to Peter Harvey whose kind advice and encouragement meant so much to me. My year in Birmingham was also enriched by the kindness of many friends there, among whom I should give special mention to the people and priests of St Francis parish, Handsworth, and some Muslim, Hindu and Marxist friends who introduced me to a wider ecumenism and helped me to appreciate the rich multi-cultural life of Birmingham.

I would also like to acknowledge the ecumenical help I have received from the different Christian churches through the secretaries of their various boards and departments dealing with issues of social responsibility and community affairs. In particular, I would like to thank Prebendary John Gladwin (Church of England), Revd Gerald M Burt (Methodist Church), Revd Donald D Black (Baptist Union of Great Britain and Ireland), Revd John Reardon (United Reform Church), Dr Isobel K Grigor (Church of Scotland), Brian V Davies (Church in Wales) and Revd Dr Stephen Orchard (British Council of Churches).

I also owe a special word of thanks to my own Archbishop, Derek Worlock. Before the project of this book had even formed in my mind, he made it possible for me to accept The Queen's College Fellowship for the year. Finally, I am deeply grateful to the people of Skelmersdale who were most understanding and generous in letting me relinquish my pastoral responsibility as team leader in the Skelmersdale Team Ministry. Although I felt I had to leave Skelmersdale if I was to continue my work as a moral theologian, it was not an easy decision to make and the parting was deeply felt on both sides. Knowing that the people of Skelmersdale understood and appreciated my decision made the parting bearable. Without their understanding I would not have had the peace of mind to write this book.

Throughout the book I have generally used the term 'embryo' to refer to all the stages of development from conception until birth. Although this is a loose usage of medical terminology, it makes for simpler reading and does not affect the substantial discussion in any way. I have also used the normal abbreviations common in the field of reproductive medicine — IVF (in-vitro fertilisation), AIH (artificial insemination with the husband's semen) and AID (artificial insemination with donor semen). Although my research has involved me in extensive reading, I have tried to make the book more readable by not using any footnotes. Quotations are identified by author, year of publication and page, with fuller details given in the bibliography. I concluded the introduction to my previous book, *Divorce and Second Marriage,* (Collins,1982), by stating: 'Reluctantly I have accepted traditional usage and used 'he' in an indefinite sense. Does justice oblige me to use 'she' in the same way if I ever write another book on this subject?' (p.17) As it has turned out, the subject matter of this book has made it easier to avoid using either 'he' or 'she' in a generic sense. I hope I have not used any sexist language, apart from its unavoidable inclusion in passages quoted from other sources.

1

What the churches are saying about IVF

What the different churches say about the morality of IVF as currently practised will depend, to a large extent, on how they interpret the status of the embryo. This will be the theme of Chapter 3. The present chapter focuses on IVF viewed precisely as a method of human procreation. The first question it faces is: prescinding from the fate of surplus embryos, do the churches accept IVF *in principle* as a method of human procreation? Moreover, since all the churches acknowledge a God-given link between procreation and marriage, there is a second question which must also be faced in this chapter. It is this: even if the churches are prepared to view IVF as ethically acceptable in principle, how do they react to IVF when it includes some form of donor-involvement?

I Is IVF acceptable in principle?

The position of most churches — IVF is acceptable in principle

Apart from the Roman Catholic Church, all the churches whose statements on IVF I have been able to study arrive at a favourable judgement *in principle* regarding IVF. They see no moral objection to IVF as a procedure, although some churches have reservations about how this procedure may actually work in practice. Examples of the kind of positions adopted are:

THE CHURCH OF ENGLAND

> 'The responsible use of IVF to remove the disability of childlessness within marriage will not threaten to undermine the interweaving of procreational and relational goods in general within marriage. In fact, in specific marriages, it may offer an enrichment of the marriage relationship which both partners gladly accept.' (*Personal Origins*, n.106)

THE FREE CHURCH FEDERAL COUNCIL AND
THE BRITISH COUNCIL OF CHURCHES

'*In vitro* fertilisation of a woman's ovum by her husband's sperm, and implantation of the embryo at a suitable time in her womb, in principle pose no moral problems. They are an extension of AIH. In practice, however, a moral objection arises if this procedure involves unjustifiable risk to the future life and well-being of the human being conceived in this way. The risk ought not to be greater than that involved in normal processes of conception and birth.' (*Choices in Childlessness*, pp.54-55, cf. also p.47)

THE BAPTIST UNION OF GREAT BRITAIN

'There seem to be no critical moral objections to this technique, together with embryo-transfer, where the ovum and sperm of a married couple are involved. Contrary factors would be: (a) the danger as with any genetic manipulation of treating human life as mere genetic material; (b) the question of the cost of the process in the light of just distribution of resources. But in many situations these factors could be outweighed by the benefit of relieving the pain of childlessness, and the responsibility of man to co-operate with God in the enrichment of life.' (*Evidence*, p.8)

THE CHURCH OF SCOTLAND

'As a technique to relieve infertility within the husband/wife relationship, IVF raises no moral questions. However, when superovulation is used to produce more embryos than will be transferred to the mother's uterus, questions arise concerning the deliberate creation of new life without hope of its potential being realised.' (p.290, n.6)

Why IVF is acceptable

What sort of analysis has led to this clear consensus among most of the churches in favour of IVF?

Christians believe that marriage is a God-given human institution. The will of God can be clearly discerned in its basic 'goods'. *Personal Origins* spells out the 'goods' of marriage:

'The union of two people in the completeness of marriage involving sexual, social, emotional and relational aspects, is seen as promoting three central goods of human life: namely, the transmission of life in the human community, a disciplined structure of living in which the individual may grow to moral maturity, and a strong and enduring relationship between them. In short we may speak of the "procreational", "moral" and "relational" goods of marriage.' (n.99)

Since the procreation of children is one of the 'goods' of marriage, Christians will naturally welcome ways to remedy childlessness in marriage. Such remedies will enable married couples to live and enjoy the fulness of their marriage in all its three 'goods'.

The Christian view of marriage does not view its different 'goods' as entirely separate from each other. They are intimately related. Christians do not see it as a mere accident of evolution that it is the act of 'making love' which can initiate the life-giving process leading to the conception and eventual birth of a new human person. Children are seen as the 'fruit' of married love. Married love is 'life-giving' love. As well as empowering the couple to live more fully themselves, it also has the potentiality to create new human beings to share in their parents' love and to grow and develop themselves as loving persons. That is why the 'life-giving' role of the parents' love is not restricted to 'giving life' in the sense of 'conceiving and giving birth to a new life'. The whole process of nurturing and education is an equally essential part of 'giving life'. The whole climate of being wanted, of trust and acceptance, created by the parents' love in the home is crucial if children are to be given life in the full sense of the word — that is, if they are to grow and develop as persons able to love and be loved. It is in this very full sense that the Christian view of marriage believes that the procreational and relational goods of marriage should be held together. That is why, at least in principle, it welcomes any new development which can render fertile a marriage which is deprived of the procreational good.

The artificiality of the process is no objection

In exploring the ethics of IVF the fundamental issue which can give rise to concern is not the 'artificiality' of the process. What is artificial will normally be welcomed as good insofar as it remedies some natural deficiency or even improves on what is natural. Ethical question-marks only begin to appear when it is thought that an artificial procedure might in fact be having a dehumanising effect. Then, however, it is the alleged 'inhumanity' of the process that gives cause for concern, not its artificiality. There will be few Christians who would disagree with the position of *Choices in Childlessness* regarding the relationship between what is 'artificial' and what is 'human':

'. . . the popular ethical distinction between the "natural" and the "unnatural" is a distinction between what is in keeping with human nature and what is not. It is not a distinction between the natural and artificial. Since, then, human beings are by nature intelligent and creative, and the adaptation of the environment to their needs is an expression of their intelligence, human artifice, such as that developed in medical technology, is in principle ethically natural. It is a mistake to condemn some piece of medical intervention as "unnatural" simply because it is artificial and sophisticated. On the other hand, the ethical distinction between the natural and the unnatural does recognise that there are limits beyond which human intervention ought not to go. These limits are transgressed when such intervention renders our humanity less than human. Where and what these limits are in any specific case is matter for moral assessment and judgment.' (p.42)

Therefore, if there is an objection to be faced regarding IVF, it will not be because it is 'artificial'. It can only be because some people consider it 'inhuman'.

Holding together the procreational and relational 'goods' of marriage

Can it be argued that IVF is 'inhuman' because it fails to hold together sufficiently the procreational and relational 'goods' of marriage by separating procreation from the human act of intercourse? The question of holding together the procreational and relational 'goods' is usually discussed in the context of contraception. Does that discussion throw any light on how these two 'goods' might be held together in the case of IVF?

The Church of England and other Christian churches have argued that, even when contraceptives are used, the procreational and relational 'goods' of marriage are still held together in a loving marriage. That is because these two 'goods' inspire the couple's whole relationship. They devote themselves to each other and to their children. Consequently, it is precisely within the couple's marriage relationship itself that these two 'goods' are held together essentially. *Personal Origins* states:

> '. . . the important points are: that procreation should not occur entirely outside the loving relationship; and that the loving relationship should issue in the good of children, unless there are strong reasons to the contrary (like genetic defect of a grave kind).' (n.103)

However, it is not essential that this 'holding together' of the procreational and relational 'goods' of marriage be fully expressed symbolically in every single act of intercourse. Even contraceptive intercourse is still truly 'life-giving' as well as loving, since it expresses and deepens the couple's life-giving love for each other and their family.

Personal Origins sees this line of argument as relevant to its discussion of IVF. It argues that if the use of contraceptives does not violate the essential 'holding together' of the procreational and relational goods of marriage, neither does the use of artificial techniques of procreation. 'As long as such techniques are not used entirely outside the context of a loving relationship' their use can be justified by an extension of this same line of argument; and the report continues: '. . . in such cases, the technique is offered as an aid to the restoration of a good proper to the marriage, which through some handicap has been impeded. So it is calculated to strengthen the relational good, and the bond between the various goods which go together to make a proper Christian marriage.' (p.37) It is this line of argument which enables *Personal Origins* to conclude finally:

> 'A Christian couple may decide that, if it is permissible to plan responsibly the number and timing of children, by the use of contraceptives, then we are already seeking and achieving a greater mastery over the processes of reproduction without reducing anything to the status of an object. They will know that it is not true that in each act of sexual intercourse they engender children as well as delighting in each other. And so they will not hesitate in situations where they are not otherwise able to have children of their own to engender children by artificial means, within the context of their own loving relationship. They will certainly wish to guard against any undermining of commitment to the goods of marriages which, they believe, have been willed by God himself. Yet the responsible use of IVF to remove the disability of childlessness within marriage will not threaten to undermine the interweaving of procreational and relational goods in general within marriage. In fact, in specific marriages, it may offer an enrichment of the marriage relationship which both partners gladly accept.' (n.106)

I have been outlining the argument in favour of IVF as it is presented in the Church of England report, *Personal Origins*. That is because, on this aspect of the matter, it develops the line of argument more thoroughly than do the reports of the other church bodies. However, my impression is that its main line of argument would be acceptable to the other Christian churches who are able to accept the prior position that the relational and procreational goods of marriage are adequately 'kept together' when contraceptive measures are employed to prevent particular acts of intercourse being open to procreation. Since this approach believes that the holding together of the procreational and relational 'goods' is situated more essentially in the loving relationship within marriage than in the act of intercourse expressing this relationship, it is able to accommodate an artificially produced conception as long as it is still within the confines of the marriage relationship itself.

The Roman Catholic position

The Roman Catholic church is in fundamental disagreement with the other churches as regards their acceptance of responsible contraception within marriage. It maintains that the relational and procreational 'goods' are not adequately kept together when the openness of the sexual act to procreation is deliberately impeded. If *Personal Origins* is correct in its judgement that the argument in favour of IVF is related to the same basic issue which underlies the argument in favour of responsible contraception, one would expect the Roman Catholic position to have some objections to IVF. In fact, the position is not quite as clear-cut as that.

An objection is certainly raised and it is elaborated at length in the evidence submitted to the Warnock Committee by the Catholic Bishops' Joint Committee on Bio-Ethical Issues speaking on behalf of the Roman Catholic Bishops of Great Britain. The argumentation underlying this objection is found in Part III of their evidence under the heading, *Possible Moral and Social Implications*. It should be stressed that this section of the Joint Committee's Evidence acknowledges that it 'includes arguments which go beyond definitive Catholic teaching' and it claims no greater authority than that 'it represents an approach favoured by most of the Joint Committee'. (n.19) We are not told why some of the Committee did not favour this approach. However, I have been reliably informed that 'the minority did not find the "product" argument a convincing reason for rejecting IVF; they did not regard accepting IVF as incompatible with *Humanae Vitae's* teaching on contraception'. It would appear that this minority view is shared by the bishops of England and Wales. There is no reason to believe that, as a body, they do not stand firmly behind the teaching of *Humanae Vitae*. Yet at the end of their November 1984 meeting they concluded a statement on the Warnock Report with the remark that 'they see no reason to consider "the simple case" of IVF as morally unacceptable.' (*Briefing*, 23/11/84, p.6) What they mean by 'the simple case', as explained in an explanatory note attached to their statement, is the case in which the sperm and egg are obtained from the husband and wife respectively and not from a third party (or 'donor') and no intentional destruction of embryos is involved. To forestall possible misunderstandings a further 'clarification' was issued shortly afterwards:

> 'The bishops did not give approval to the present practice of *in vitro* fertilisation within marriage. This they consider to be unacceptable because the process involves the intentional destruction of human embryos.

The bishops recognised that there are also serious questions about the compatibility of these practices with the Church's teaching concerning marital intercourse as the proper context for the transmission of human life. Their intention was not to engage in a comprehensive treatment of questions at this stage but to exercise prudent discernment in an area full of complex possibilities and far-reaching pastoral implications.

The bishops did not wish to exclude the possibility that future developments in *in vitro* fertilisation could eliminate those factors which make current practice immoral.' (*Briefing*, 14/12/84, p.3)

Neither the 'minority' of the Joint Committee nor the Bishops' Conference have issued any official documentation laying out the argumentation in favour of their position. Consequently, it seems best to leave aside consideration of this division of opinion until Chapter 6. For the present, therefore, it would seem more in line with the methodology I am following to examine more closely the objection raised against IVF by the 'majority' of the Catholic Bishops' Joint Committee on Bio-Ethical Issues.

IVF makes a child's relationship to its parents one of 'product' to 'makers'

The Committee do not argue from the intentions of the IVF parents. In fact, far from presuming any unworthy motives on the part of the parents, they actually envisage them to be acting from the highest motivation —

'. . . we have been envisaging parents whose motives are good motives, whose desire to have a child of their own is human and good, whose choice of IVF had none of the serious wrongfulness of choices against human life in being or human life in its transmission, and whose subsequent dedication in nurturing and educating their child together may well enhance and strengthen their marital relationship.' (n.27)

Instead, their argument is founded on what they consider to be the in-built significance of the IVF process and the effect that this will inevitably have on the IVF parents themselves, despite their highest motivation.

'To choose to have a child by IVF is to choose to have a child as the product of a making. But the relationship of product to maker is a relationship of radical inequality, of profound subordination. Thus the choice to have or to create a child by IVF is a choice in which the child does not have the status which the child of sexual union has, a status which is a great good for any child: the status of radical equality with parents, as partner like them in the familial community.' (n.25)

The key lies in the intrinsic meaning of sexual intercourse

The flaw they see in the IVF process lies precisely in the separation of pro-creation from sexual intercourse. The conjunction of the two is needed if the child is to come into existence as an equal partner in the life of the couple —

> '(24) . . . the IVF child comes into existence, not as a gift supervening on an act expressive of marital union, and so not in the manner of a new partner in the common life so vividly expressed by that act, but rather in the manner of a pro-duct of a making (and indeed, typically, as the end-product of a process managed and carried out by persons other than his parents). . .

> (26) . . . The act of sexual intercourse profoundly embodies, expresses and enacts this submission to membership in a partnership. In this respect there is a profound difference between procreation by intercourse, even an act of inter-course which the spouses hope and expect will result in procreation. Such an act, even if engaged in at a time calculated by them most likely to be fertile, will properly be an act inherently expressive of the marital partnership and thus quite different from any human acts of making, producing or acquiring a pos-session. Freely chosen by the spouses, it has nonetheless a physical and emo-tional structure making it inherently apt to be experienced by each partner as a giving of self and receiving of the other, a giving which may be complemented by the gift of a child. That gift of a child will have come, then, not from any act of mastery, even jointly agreed mastery, over extraneous materials, even natural biological materials. Rather, the child will have come from an act of mutual involvement between persons (involvement at all levels, physical, emotional, intelligent and moral).
> In thus giving and submitting themselves each to the other, these partners in marriage are opening themselves up (and submitting themselves) both to the profound source of life from which the child (they hope) can come, and to ser-vice of the child and of each other in the unforeseeable contingencies of their new role as parents . . . That . . . is why the child of such a union, although weak and dependent, enters the community of the family not as an object of produc-tion but as a kind of *partner* in the familial enterprise; and as such this child has a fundamental *parity or equality with the parents.*' (nn.24 & 26)

The proponents of this view state their position very moderately. They recognise that good IVF parents will try to avoid the danger they are high-lighting but they see this as a deeper issue than mere good-will. 'If the par-ents are to be good parents, they will strive to assign the child his or her true status as a member of the human race and of their own family. But in so doing, they will be labouring against the real structure of the decisive choices and against the deep symbolism of all that was done to bring that child into being.' (n.27) Their final conclusion is not expressed in terms of an absolutist prohibition of IVF but as a warning against the harmful consequences of the 'logic' of radical domination involved in IVF and against its 'morally flawed procedures, which inherently undermine fundamental human good and the attitudes appropriate to it.' (n.27)

Similar positions outside the Roman Catholic church

Many people right across the spectrum of the Christian churches and beyond have reservations about IVF which are at least remotely linked to the separation of procreation from intercourse. These reservations concern the effect that IVF might be having on our perception and appreciation of parenthood. Such reservations need not lead to an absolutist stance against IVF. Remedying infertility is good and IVF can be welcomed insofar as it is a form of infertility therapy. The reservations are focused more on the possibility of a new 'norm' of parenthood becoming accepted, as advances in reproductive technology open out new styles of parenthood to parents or even to single women, and possibly even to single men.

A line of argument which has a certain affinity to the 'majority' position of the Roman Catholic committee is mentioned in the Church of England Board of Social Responsibility Report, *Personal Origins* (1985), n.105 —

'It is thought that we may be attempting to achieve a mastery over human nature itself, possibly involving a reduction of it to the status of an object to be made and manipulated, in encouraging a technological way of thinking about procreation. The natural processes embody and express much larger patterns and relationships on which our whole experience of the world and each other depends . . . What is feared is the impact on our culture of a technological way of thinking about sexual intercourse and procreation. Those who feel this strongly will be reluctant to embark on such a procedure. They feel that sexual intercourse forms the centre of a network of instinctive family relationships which is complex and deep-rooted, and that nothing should be countenanced which threatens this complex network.' (p.38)

It is not clear whether any on the Committee would identify themselves with this position. The previous paragraph has already stated that for anyone who accepts 'the permissibility — and indeed the desirability — of sundering procreative and relational acts in particular cases', there is no problem about the artificiality of IVF in marriage since it is 'an aid to the restoration of a good proper to the marriage, which through some handicap has been impeded.' There is nothing to suggest that all the Committee do not agree with this. In fact, even their statement of the 'human technology' objection seems to say that this will have no harmful effect on a rightly-motivated couple. 'It is clearly possible for a mature and thoughtful couple to use a technical procedure in procreation without coming to think any differently about each other and about their children than they would otherwise have done.' (n.105) Were the *Personal Origins* Committee, therefore, merely voicing a view which they recognised to be peculiar to the Roman Catholic Church or was there some sympathy for this view on the Committee itself? The evidence would seem to suggest that the latter is true.

One of the members of the Committee responsible for *Personal Origins* was Professor Oliver O'Donovan. His book, *Begotten or Made?* (Oxford University Press, 1984), leads me to think that he might have been mainly responsible for the inclusion of n.105 in *Personal Origins*. O'Donovan discusses IVF specifically in Chapter 5 of *Begotten or Made?*, though his general remarks in Chapter 1 are very relevant. Although he cannot accept the Roman Catholic Joint Committee's position since it puts too much emphasis on the *act* of sexual intercourse rather than on the over-all sexual relationship, yet he shares their fear about the 'product' mentality. Clearly, therefore, in O'Donovan's mind the Roman Catholic 'product' argument is not inseparably bound up with its position on the holding together of the procreational and relational 'goods' of marriage in 'the one intentional act' of intercourse. Moreover, O'Donovan believes that the embryo enjoys an equal status with any other human being. Hence, he regards IVF as seriously flawed because it has developed from and is still dependent on experimental research on embryos and also because it involves being prepared to take unknown risks with human beings. O'Donovan concludes his examination of the issue of IVF by expressing a concern very akin to the Roman Catholic Report and n.105 of *Personal Origins*:

> 'I confess that I do not know how to think of an IVF child except (in some unclear but inescapable sense) as the *creature* of the doctors who assisted at her conception — which means, also, of the society to which the doctor belongs and for whom he acts.
>
> . . . If our habits of thought continue to instruct us that the IVF child is radically equal to the doctors who produced her, then that is good — for the time being. But if we do not live and act in accordance with such conceptions, and if society welcomes more and more institutions and practices which implicitly deny them, then they will soon appear to be merely sentimental, the tatters and

shreds which remind us of how we used once to clothe the world with intelligibility.' (pp.85-86)

Is the IVF child the fruit of its parents' love?

Could the objection we have been examining be expressed more simply as: the IVF child is not the fruit of its parents' love. Although it may have had its origin in an instinctive feeling of that kind, such a simple statement does not do justice to the far more sophisticated version of the objection presented, for instance, by the Roman Catholic Bishops' Bioethical Committee. In fact, it is probably accepted by most people nowadays, even those opposed to IVF, that it is precisely the infertile couple's mutual love and their desire to share that love which drives them to seek a child by IVF. It could even be said that their actual decision to try to have an IVF child is itself an expression of their love. Their willingness to undergo both personal and material hardship to have a child is a clear indication of how self-sacrificing their love is prepared to be. It is probably true to say that an IVF baby is likely to be even more a 'wanted' baby than a child conceived normally. The fact that the IVF child is not the fruit of the specific act of love which is sexual intercourse does not mean that it is in no way the fruit of its parents' love.

Although acts of sexual intercourse can express and even deepen a couple's love for each other, yet their love lies essentially in them as persons and in their relationship to one another. It is true that, for this love to stay alive and grow, they need to express it to each other in all sorts of ways. It is also true that sexual intercourse holds a special place in the language of love. Nevertheless, it still remains only one expression of love among many within marriage. Even refraining from intercourse can be an expression of love on occasion. Even the sufferings that the woman has to go through in infertility treatment and the feeling of helplessness experienced by the man throughout the process can be transformed into expressions of self-sacrificing love. The same is true of the sacrifice of creature comforts they might need to accept together to cover the costs of treatment. There are many different ways in which a couple can express their love for each other and their desire to share their mutual love with a child of their own. Any children they have are the fruit of that love and not simply of specific acts expressing that love.

The Roman Catholic Report does not doubt that the IVF couple are motivated by love; rather it expresses the fear that the IVF process will inevitably have an eroding effect on their love. Despite their best intentions the IVF process is such that they will experience their child as a 'product'. They provide the raw materials, as it were, but the crucial stages of the process are controlled by people extrinsic to their relationship. Though these 'third parties' are genuinely committed to helping the couple with their infertility problem, the very nature of the process with its in-built canons of efficiency and quality-control creates a climate in which much of the wonder of new life is lost and in which the quality of the life produced becomes predominant. Unconsciously, so the argument goes, the couple will be looking for a 'good quality' baby which the technicians, acting as third parties, will produce from the selection of embryos available to them. This almost imperceptible shift to 'quality' thinking will inevitably put at risk the total and unconditional acceptance of a child by its parents which would seem to be the one essential pre-requisite if a child is to grow and develop in the secure family atmosphere created by its parents' love. Without any specifically Christian point of reference, this argument is put very forcefully by Barbara Katz Rothman —

> 'Parenthood demands such total acceptance from us. We expect mothers to love, to accept their babies unreservedly, with the fullness of their hearts, no matter what. We joke about: "A face only a mother could love". It is not that women have always been able to achieve that unconditional love. Indeed, the fear of having a child one cannot love is one of the more common fears that haunt pregnancy. But never before have we asked women to make rational, intellectual determinations based on that fear. What does it do to motherhood, to women, and to men as fathers too, when we make parental acceptance conditional, pending further testing? We ask the mother and her family to say, in essence, "These are my standards. If you meet these standards of acceptability, then you are mine and I will love and accept you totally. After you pass this test."' (Rothman 1985, p.190)

It is this totally accepting love, it is claimed, that is threatened by IVF and other processes in reproductive technology.

Whose needs does IVF serve — the parents' or the children's?

The Roman Catholic position as found in the Evidence to the Warnock Committee from the Bishops' Joint Committee on Bioethical Issues insists that the needs of the children are primary. It is not sufficient that prospective parents want to have children. Their desire for children is unreasonable if the situation into which the child will be born is likely to be harmful to the child's personal development:

'. . . children have the right to have been brought into the world in the context which tends best to promote their individuality and responsibility and their sense of identity, and which characteristically affords them the most all-round and discriminating support in the crises of development and even of later life . . .' (n.16)

In their Response to the *Warnock Report* the Joint Committee make this one of their major objections. They argue that the Warnock Commission has subordinated the interests of the prospective child to the interests of the adults involved:

'The interests of embryo and child, i.e. of the new human being who is either being envisaged and planned for or who actually exists, are systematically subordinated to the interests of the adults who (very understandably) want a child. And those interests and rights of the newly generated are subordinated to the optimisation of a technique for fulfilling that adult want.' (n.11)

The other Christian churches are not inattentive to the needs of the children, especially since they 'are unable to look after their own interests for themselves'. (*Choices in Childlessness*, p.20) However, they believe that the deepest interests of the children are inseparably linked to the love and stability of the marriage itself. Hence, they refuse to isolate the welfare of the children from 'the good of Christian marriage'. (*Personal Origins*, p.113) The interests of the parents and the interests of the children are mutually dependent each on the other.

It could be argued that the difference of emphasis here between the Roman Catholic position we have been examining and the other Christian churches comes back to the same key issue which has been high-lighted in this chapter. The other Christian churches emphasise the importance of the parents' relationship for the good of the children and in that sense locate the holding together of the relational and the procreational 'goods' essentially in the relationship itself. The Roman Catholic position does not accept that. Consequently, it is more inclined to think that 'because the parents want a child' is a reason which only looks to the parents' needs and not one which will normally be answering the future child's needs as well.

Why is there such a major difference between the Roman Catholic position and the other Christian churches on this issue of whether within marriage the holding together of the procreational and the relational 'goods' occurs essentially in the act of sexual intercourse or in the couple's relationship of life-giving love? That question will be examined further in Chapter 2.

II   Is IVF *with donor involvement acceptable? The intrusion of third parties into the marriage relationship and parenthood*

The third parties under consideration here are the donors of sperm or ova or embryos and surrogate mothers or women who are prepared to carry in their womb a child which is not their own. While it is true that third parties can also take the form of the medical personnel and scientists involved in the IVF procedures, the possible impact of their involvement has already been touched on in the previous section.

Some questions raised by donor involvement in IVF

The involvement of a third-party as donor in IVF raises a number of questions for the Christian churches:

(1) Does third party involvement offend against the exclusive character of the marriage relationship? Is it a new form of adultery?

(2) When donor sperm or donor ova are used, does the non-contributing partner feel alienated by the process and does this seriously affect his or her sense of being a true parent of the child? Is this likely to be a greater difficulty for the father in the case of sperm-donation, if he feels reduced to the role of a non-involved on-looker throughout the whole process?

(3) Since donor involvement creates a situation of multi-parentage (with greater or lesser complexity, depending on the circumstances), is this exposing the resulting child to the danger of a major psychological crisis regarding personal identity and all the harmful consequences flowing from this?

(4) Does the process foster an attitude of genetic irresponsibility on the part of donors?

How do the various Christian Churches respond to these questions?

THE CHURCH OF ENGLAND

The Anglican Board for Social Responsibility has twice expressed itself on the question of donor involvement since the publication of the *Warnock Report*. The first occasion was when it published its Response to the *Warnock Report*. In this Response, while acknowledging that the contrary position had previously been the 'official' teaching of the Church of England, it expressed a strong majority position accepting AID and argued its case as follows:

> 'AID introduces a third party into the intimacies of married life. Marriage is the union of one man and one woman for life. The Memorandum of Evidence submitted on this issue in 1959 on behalf of the Church of England reaffirmed the finding of the Archbishop of Canterbury's Commission of 1948 that "artificial insemination with donated semen involves a breach of the marriage. It violates the exclusive union set up between husband and wife" (n.3, p.58). There are those who hold that when a couple become 'one flesh' in marriage, they belong to one another in such a close and exclusive way that nothing and no one else should take their place both in sexual union and in the procreation that normally results from it. For such people union and procreation are indissolubly linked. There can be, however, a proper development of Anglican ethical thinking on matters concerning sex (cf. the development of Anglican thinking on contraception). It is possible for a couple today to hold in good conscience the conviction that the semen of a third party imports nothing alien into the marriage relationship and does not adulterate it as physical union would. It is a possible view of the exclusiveness of the marital relationship that it concerns physical congress rather than the giving and reception of semen which is its normal accompaniment. *The majority of us agree with the Report that "those engaging in AID are, in their own view, involved in a positive affirmation of the family" (4.14) and hence AID may be regarded as an acceptable practice.'*
> (5.2)

The Board for Social Responsibility spoke again on this issue in its more comprehensive report on human fertilisation and embryology entitled *Personal Origins* (1985). This report acknowledges that gamete donation (i.e. donation of sperm and/or ova) has certain features which are in common with adoption and certain features in common with adultery. Yet all its members agree that it should not be equated with either. Unlike adoption, the prospective parents' decision is not about an already existing child. Theirs is a 'much more consciously responsible role'. (n.108) They are actually deciding to bring a child into existence. Although the child is not genetically their own as a couple, the situation is very different from adultery since 'there is no breaking of the relationship of physical fidelity and there is no real relationship with a person outside the marriage'. (n.109) Nevertheless, there is a problem here that divides the Committee. They all recognise that in gamete donation 'procreation is separated from relationship completely, at the genetic level, even though the connection between the two is preserved at the social level' (n.107) but they cannot agree about how morally significant this is —

> 'We differ on this, depending on whether we see the genetic as the most basic manifestation of the personal and find the alienation of genetic parenthood from marriage a development which undermines the Christian understanding; or whether we judge that, although everyone is fundamentally influenced and limited by his or her genetic endowment, nevertheless the overriding factor is the social context which can assure proper love, respect and care. To this extent the question of genetic origin is not of fundamental moral importance, when compared with the question of how the child will be loved and cared for.' (n.109)

The Committee also divide on whether the 'dominion over nature' problem is further aggravated by the introduction of a donor element. To some it 'introduces an element of dominion over nature which appears unjustifiable . . . and possibly even threatening to human values'. (n.110) To others it is simply a further extension of responsible control over procreation and any dangers involved should be coped with by appropriate safeguards rather than by prohibition.

However, the Committee are in full agreement over their practical rejection of surrogate motherhood — 'In surrogate motherhood the Christian institution of the family is fundamentally endangered, and thus. . . it cannot be morally acceptable as a practice for Christians'. (n.112)

In the final analysis it is not easy to determine where precisely *Personal Origins* stands on the basic issue of donor involvement. For instance, it repeats almost verbatim the whole passage from n.5.2 of the Response to the *Warnock Report* quoted on page 29 above. Yet very significantly it omits the final sentence in that quotation. In its chapter headed *Conclusions for Practice* it admits that it has been divided as a Working Party but, unlike in the Response, no indication is given as to the relative numerical strength of support for the two positions.

> 'Nature is God-given, but is flawed. Human beings are called to co-operate with God in treating and (so far as possible) remedying any natural deficiency. We gratefully acknowledge the blessings that come from a right use of medical technology to assist a couple in founding a family. In considering embryo donation we have had to determine the boundaries beyond which we should not transgress in altering the course of nature. We have found here, as we have experienced elsewhere, a theological division concerning the extent to which nature is given by God with its ends determined, and the extent to which we may regard it as 'raw material' to fashion for our own good ends. Some would

argue, particularly in the case of embryo donation, that technological interference with the course of nature goes far beyond the remedying of a natural defect. They believe that the fertilisation of an ovum by artificial means from an anonymous donor, to be implanted in a mother and reared by parents who have no genetic relationship with the child, entails treating that child too much as a product. Opponents of the practice fear that knowledge about his or her totally anonymous origins might have a deleterious effect on a person born in this way. Nevertheless, the distinction between implanting an embryo with a donated ovum, one with donated semen, and one where both ovum and semen are donated, seems one of degree. Once the principle of donation is granted, some would see little reason to insist that at least 50 per cent of the embryo's genes should be those of one social parent. When genetic and social parentage have been sundered in principle, it seems an uneasy compromise to try to reaffirm a partial link between the two.' (n.125)

Perhaps the most accurate statement of the Working Party's final stance on donor involvement is the following:

'Finally, we would wish to reiterate that our fundamental concern in these matters is for the preservation of the good of Christian marriage, as instituted by God himself, and for the welfare of children, who are to be brought up in the fear and love of the Lord. It will need much observation and discussion before we can come to a clear mind about whether these practices threaten marriage or the true welfare of children, or conversely if they are a blessing in marriage. But it is above all important to recognise the new situation in which we stand, with possibilities now open to us which have never before existed. In this situation, our traditions of moral thought need to be extended and rethought. It may well be that previous ways of thinking will not be sustainable on reflection. On the other hand, we should not give up too lightly positions which have been important to generations of Christians.' (n.113)

THE FREE CHURCH FEDERAL COUNCIL AND THE BRITISH COUNCIL OF CHURCHES

The British Council of Churches and Free Church Council Report, *Choices in Childlessness* (1982), also admits to a division of views among its members. Their division is concerned with whether or not the involvement of a donor violates the exclusivity of the marriage covenant.

'Some of us from the outset took the view, from which no further argument or reflection dislodged us, that there is a specifically Christian objection to the practice of AID. This rested on the conviction that marriage is a covenant-relationship between husband and wife exclusive of all others, not only in sexual intercourse, but also in the procreation of children. If there is going to be a child by the one, then so long as the covenant relationship endures, it shall be a child by both; if it is not to be by both, then it shall be by neither. This is part of the meaning of marriage 'for better, for worse'. A covenant-relationship of this kind does not, of course, rule out adoption, but it rules out AID as much as it rules out adultery.

Others of us took the view that the full and informed consent to AID of both husband and wife materially altered the case. Such consent cannot in principle be invalidated by the existence of a covenant-relationship. It can be incorporated within the covenant and may in certain circumstances support and even strengthen it.' (p.43)

The Report also expresses 'anxiety' over the possible harmful effects of gamete donation on the resulting child's sense of personal identity, linking this with such practical questions as mixing donor and husband sperm and the anonymity of the donor.

'Ancestry may not be altogether irrelevant to identity. If our primary concern is really for the interests of the child, we should be sure that the risks to which we are subjecting an AID child are not substantially greater than the risks to which we should be willing to subject any other child. So far we do not have the evidence necessary for making reliable comparisons.' (p.44)

Like *Personal Origins* the BCC-Free Church Report is in no doubt about its condemnation of surrogate motherhood —

'The surrrogate mother . . . provides more than the ovum . . . (She) has . . . a deepening relationship which, begun before birth, would in the normal course of events be expected to continue after birth. Deliberately to disrupt this relationship is totally to alter its character and to damage its potentiality. It is to act irresponsibly and inhumanly. It is to reduce procreation to nothing more than a biological process. Surrogate motherhood is hardly motherhood at all.' (p.48)

The final conclusion of *Choices in Childlessness* is far more against than in favour of any donor involvement — 'Although, as a group, we are not prepared to condemn AID outright, nevertheless we are sufficiently impressed by the objections raised against it to wish to register our disquiet, and call for a public inquiry.' (p.45)

THE ROMAN CATHOLIC CHURCH

Donor involvement in all forms is regarded as morally unacceptable by the Roman Catholic Bishops' Joint Committee on Bio-Ethical Issues. They state the principle that 'children have a right to be born the true child of a married couple, and thus to have an unimpaired sense of identity'. (n.17, p.11) Their position is clearly based on what they see to be in the best interests of the prospective child. 'The rights and interests of the prospective child. . . should systematically prevail over the understandable desires of men or women who want a child.' (n.18, p.11) Nevertheless, they are careful to state that this line of argument does not justify abortion, once conception has taken place. 'Even when the cause of their conception involved serious wrong-doing or unwisdom, children once conceived are not "better off dead".' (n.17, p.11)

THE CHURCH OF SCOTLAND

The Church of Scotland, likewise, is opposed to any form of donor involvement and sees 'in AID the unwarranted intrusion of a third party in the marriage relationship, which it cannot support'. (p.290) Hence, it states: 'Profound as feelings associated with infertility unquestionably are, the experience of infertility should not be taken to advocate practices such as AID, embryo transfer or egg donation which imply either the introduction of a third party into the marriage relationship or treat women as merely incubators or men as disinterested donors of sperm.' (p.289)

THE BAPTIST UNION OF GREAT BRITAIN AND IRELAND

One of the clearest and most thorough moral considerations of donor involvement is that found in the evidence submitted to the Warnock Committee on behalf of the Baptist Union of Great Britain and Ireland. Regarding AID they list the 'strong contrary factors which a Christian ethic would urge' —

'(a) the use of unknown sperm or ova intensifies the tendency to treat human genetic material as objects to be manipulated, and even sold commercially, rather than as the basis for personality. There are dangerous implications for social awareness here:
(b) the use of unknown sperm or ova means that the procreator has no responsibility for his/her offspring. The conception of children is thus divorced from the context of responsible relationships. While this may unfortunately happen in other circumstances in which a child is conceived normally, here it is built into the process as an inevitable element;
(c) the use of sperm and ova "banks" encourages the selection of certain genetic types as "desirable" and opens the door to a programme of positive eugenics. This is offensive to Christian morality, which believes that God gives value to human life rather than man;

(d) the child is deprived of the right to know the identity of its father/mother. While this may happen in normal instances of conception, here again it is built into the process;

(e) while AID or egg-donation could hardly be defined as "adultery" or "unfaithfulness" within the Christian ethic, it does disturb the principle of "one flesh" within Christian marriage, where sexual union is understood to be the active symbol of a covenantal relationship.'

In the light of the above 'strong contrary factors' the conclusion drawn is: 'A Christian ethic would be likely to resist the development of AID and egg-donation as a normally available method for overcoming infertility. Supporting factors would have to be very strong indeed to outweigh the contrary ones.' (n.13)

The Baptist Union evidence also gives a similar list of 'strong contrary factors' against the practice of womb leasing —

'(a) the surrogate mother is treated as a mere incubator, ignoring the effect upon her personality and physiology of carrying and bearing a child. . .

(b) the foetus is also being regarded as less than a potential personality, ignoring the interaction between mother and child in the uterine stage. Stimuli from the uterine environment influence the development of the nervous system as well as probably producing feelings that may have a long-lasting effect;

(c) . . . Some psychiatrists say that the first three months of pregnancy are crucial to the psychological development of the unborn child. The mother's feelings of well-being, contentment, rejection, love or unlove, can be transferred to the foetus and remembered in his subconscious for the rest of his life. . . Although nothing is conclusive in this area, it does indicate that whereas in terms of the physical we are beginning to understand the start of life, when it comes to the psyche we still have a lot of research to do. What we are considering in this report are processes that could cause untold psychological harm;

(d) . . . in the USA . . . it is reported that frequently the surrogate mother refuses to give up the baby. . . ' (n.14)

Consequently, womb leasing is rejected by this Baptist Union report as 'normally unacceptable to a Christian ethic'.

THE CHURCH IN WALES

The Church in Wales, in their response to the *Warnock Report,* have a long section on AID. They express grave concern about 'the involvement of a "third party", an anonymous and non-responsible third person, into what ought to be an exclusive marriage covenant' but they are far from suggesting that there is anything akin to adultery in this. Far from it: when both partners fully consent to AID it could be a very rich expression of their mutual fidelity:

> 'When AID is undertaken out of such a freely-given mutual consent, when it is decided on as an act of love expressing the inner meaning of the marriage covenant, when it expresses the desire for a child of the wife's own flesh who will be the child of the parenthood covenant of the husband as well as the wife, then AID hardly constitutes adultery. To the contrary, it may well express the very opposite: fidelity in the richest sense of the term.' (p.4)

They also express concern about 'the psychological factors relating to AID'. They recognise that the husband and wife will be affected differently:

> 'Undoubtedly the husband usually has the greater psychological adjustment to make in these procedures. He is the "deficient" one, a difficult role for many in a society with exaggerated masculine virility images. The effect on the woman is not by any means less smooth. Somehow she must cope both with her husband's deficiency and with the potential guilt of carrying "another man's baby' in her womb." (p.4)

Summing up

Can we draw any final conclusion concerning the position of the various Christian churches on the moral acceptability of IVF with donor involvement?

All the questions mentioned on page 28 are considered by most of the churches. Their conclusions can be summarised as follows:

(1) No church condemns donor involvement in IVF as a form of adultery but some churches believe that it is not really in accord with the exclusivity of the marriage covenant. However, not all the churches who adopt this position would go on to draw the conclusion that AID is to be rejected in all circumstances.

(2) The possibility of the non-contributing partners feeling alienated is acknowledged but this is not viewed as a major objection to the practice. It is merely a negative factor to be borne in mind.

(3) The potential harm to the IVF child due to confusion or ambiguity over personal identity and anonymous parentage comes over as the objection which carries most weight among the churches. Nevertheless, the lack of empirical evidence needed to substantiate this objection is acknowledged.

(4) Genetic irresponsibility is acknowledged as a further contributory negative factor. There is total agreement over the rejection of surrogate motherhood or womb-leasing on the grounds that this violates the personal dignity of the woman involved and might also have harmful effects on the child.

As regards arriving at any kind of clear over-all moral evaluation, no church, among those whose statements I have been able to examine, is unreservedly in favour of IVF with donor involvement. The Roman Catholic church and the Church of Scotland are quite definite in their rejection of it. The Baptist Union also comes out against it but is less absolute in its judgement. The Church in Wales expresses serious reservations but does not arrive at any definite moral judgement on the issue. The Church of England is divided in its report, *Personal Origins*. Although it is never stated explicitly in the Report, one senses that within the Working Party it is the majority who consider that IVF with donor involvement is morally acceptable. *Choices in Childlessness,* the Report sponsored by the Free Church Federal Council and the British Council of Churches, reflects a division of opinion among its members. However, in the end they seem to lean more towards rejection than acceptance.

2

Analysing what the churches say about IVF

It is very evident from the previous chapter's analysis of the official positions of the various Christian churches that there is far from being a united front among them on the issue of IVF. This chapter will examine how far the Christian churches are agreed on the basic Christian values which provide the foundation for any assessment of the morality of IVF. At this level, as might be expected, there is virtually complete agreement. The chapter will also examine the ways in which the different churches bring these values to bear on the issue of IVF. It is here that differences become apparent. I shall try to explore why these differences occur.

Basic areas of agreement

All the Christian churches agree that any responsible use of IVF and reproductive technology must respect the 'goods' of marriage itself. These 'goods' are well summed up in a statement from *Personal Origins*:

> 'The union of two people in the completeness of marriage involving sexual, social, emotional and relational aspects, is seen as promoting three central goods of human life: namely, the transmission of life in the human community, a disciplined structure of living in which the individual may grow to moral maturity, and a strong and enduring relationship between them. In short we may speak of the "procreational', "moral' and "relational" goods of marriage. (n.99)

In other words, the moral evaluation of IVF will be dependent on its implications for (a) the good of marriage itself as an institution whose well-being is fundamental to the whole fabric of human society; (b) the good of the particular marriage involved; (c) the welfare of the prospective child.

Obviously, all the churches are committed to the over-riding principle of Christian morality which is found in the Lord's invitation to 'love one another as I have loved you'. Furthermore, they would undoubtedly accept that there is a need to work out the practical implications of that over-riding principle in the down-to-earth daily living out of married and parental love. Consequently, the churches would also agree that the basic question they have to face about IVF could be formulated as: can IVF (either in its simple form without any donor involvement or even with some kind of donor involvement) be a true expression of Christian love?

There is also agreement among the churches on the issues to be faced if that question is to be answered satisfactorily. From all their analyses they seem fairly consistent in turning their attention to four questions which are in reality sub-divisions of this main question —

(1) does IVF contradict our responsive love to God by going beyond what we discern to be the limits of human dominion placed on us by God himself?

(2) does IVF seriously harm the God-given love of the parents?

(3) is it unloving by seriously harming the child which is itself precious to God?

(4) is it unloving by harming people in general (including future generations) by causing irreparable damage to the very institution of marriage as given by God himself for the benefit of all peoples or by threatening the health and well-being of children to be born in the future?

Consequences and intrinsic meaning — two approaches to ethical reasoning

Three of the four questions mentioned above deal with the possible consequences of IVF. The other question is quite different. It focuses on the limits to our dominion over nature. The contrast between this question and the other three highlights two different emphases in trying to discern whether a particular action is good or not. One emphasis would concentrate on the consequences. A way of acting will be regarded as morally good if its beneficial consequences sufficiently outweigh any harmful consequences resulting from it. This is the consequentialist emphasis. The other emphasis concentrates on whether this way of acting is in accordance with the essential meaning of being a human person in this world. This is the essentialist emphasis. One emphasis turns the spot-light on consequences, the other on intrinsic meaning.

Looking at IVF from a consequentialist stand-point the focus will be on the harmful consequences that it is claimed will follow from these new reproductive processes. The consequentialist argument , therefore, will concentrate on such questions as: — (1) how certain is it that that these consequences will actually come about? (2) even if these consequences will certainly come about if nothing is done to prevent them, could not human ingenuity devise some way to prevent them happening? (3) even granting the undesirability of these consequences, could it not be argued that the harm caused might be more than compensated by the good achieved? To refute the consequentialist argument on purely consequentialist grounds would demand contrary empirical evidence or a convincing argument which would prove that the grounds put forward for presuming these harmful consequences are lacking in any solid foundation.

The essentialist position, in its purest form, would not be open to such lines of argument. It does not base its case on the degree of certainty or probability regarding the consequences. Its case is founded on its assertion that this way of acting is intrinsically flawed since it runs contrary to the essential nature of the persons involved. Therefore, the essentialist position claims that the wrongness of such an action lies not in its bad consequences, but in itself. It is disordered and self-contradictory. Hence, it will inevitably create further disorder in its wake and cause still more contradictions to follow. These harmful consequences will follow as surely as night follows day. That is why the essentialist position argues that good motivation is powerless to avert these harmful consequences. The only kind of contrary argument the essentialist would accept as refuting his position is one which convincingly demonstrates that his view is based on a misunderstanding of what being a human person is really about or how this way of acting relates to the essence of being human.

Discovering what it means to be human: are there limits to our dominion?

The first of the four questions posed on page 38 above ('does IVF contradict our responsive love to God by going beyond the limits of human dominion placed on us by God himself') would usually be interpreted as an essentialist question. It seems to presume that reality ('nature') carries its own built-in meaning. Human beings do not 'confer' meaning on reality; they discover and recognise the meaning of reality.

It would appear that all the churches have at least some kind of essentialist foundation for their position. None of them suggest that the world is meaningless. As will be seen later, in discussing the status of the embryo, virtually all the churches maintain that human dignity is not something human beings 'confer' on people; it is something that is recognised and accepted. Some kind of essentialist position would seem to flow from the basic Christian stance of reverence before the 'otherness' of God, from whom all reality flows and who supports it in being. *Choices in Childlessness* presents very strongly a position which would seem to be common to all the churches:

> 'There are theological aspects, too, to our discussion of limits and limitations. Human beings are created in the "image and likeness" of God. The powers they have of imagination, inventiveness, intellect and practical skill are God-given. They are to be used creatively in the service of the human community. As God's children, created in his image, men and women are to develop and use these powers as God's stewards and co-creators. They are called to exercise God-like care.
>
> Such creative, caring use of God-given powers cannot properly be exercised without limits. We have already seen how limits which are inbuilt into the order of things provide us with a framework for development and growth. In a world where we are all interdependent, and where, to use St Paul's image of the "body", each part has its own distinctive function, genuine love and care can be expressed only when each one of us, and each group in society, recognises the limits which responsibility places on power. In some situations, such as human experimentation, or the development of nuclear power, it may be right to impose strict limits for the health and well-being, not only of those immediately involved, but also of the wider community.
>
> Theologically, a recognition of limits takes us right into the heart of God, who for the sake of his creation accepts the most radical limits on himself. He takes human form, shares human experience, and suffers death on the cross. Such self-limitation is part of the mystery of the divine Love.' (p.39)

Discovering the meaning of human life and human sexuality

If there is a fundamental division between the churches, it is certainly not on whether life has a meaning. All the churches agree on that. All Christians believe that the full meaning of life is revealed only in and through Jesus Christ. In a sense, he not only *reveals* the meaning of life in its fulness; he actually is the meaning of life. However, to say that Jesus reveals and is the meaning of life in his person does not imply that we can read off that meaning simply by focusing our attention on Jesus. We still need to explore life itself in all its aspects; we still have to try to deepen our understanding of all the layers involved in the human person and in human living. The meaning we discover through all these avenues of exploration will all be part of what it means to be truly human — and so it will be part, but only part, of the meaning of Jesus himself. However, the pathway to discover these layers of meaning must pass through human exploration and experience. Jesus does not make our search redundant. He simply makes it more rewarding. What we discover through our searching will be found to have riches of meaning we never dreamed of, since in Jesus being truly human becomes an expression of being divine. Yet, despite all that, our Christian faith does not absolve us from taking our part in the human search to understand more deeply what human sexuality, marriage and parenthood are all about.

All Christians believe in the goodness of human sexuality as part of God's handiwork. As mentioned earlier, all Christians believe in the 'goods' of marriage as instituted by God himself. Humankind has come to understand and value the goods of marriage by reflecting on its experience of human sexuality. In a sense, humankind has 'discovered' marriage in this way. Christians would stress the word 'discovered'. Although the actual form that marriage takes on is very variable and is largely dependent on cultural and historical conditions, nevertheless Christians would not view marriage as a *totally* human creation, with no deeper meaning than that of a purely sociological contract. Although the essence of marriage can never be distilled in its pristine purity from its changing cultural and historical forms, there is an underlying core meaning of marriage which Christians believe is part of God's design for human living which has been 'revealed' to humankind through this process of gradual experiential discovery. In fact, its deeper implications are still being revealed today as men and women come to understand themselves even more fully as sexual beings. A fundamental question is whether the new possibilities for parenthood being opened up by the application of modern scientific technology to the reproductive processes are yet another stage in this revelatory process of human discovery.

Why churches differ — different approaches lead to different conclusions

The problem that the Christian churches are grappling with in their explorations into this issue is not simply: what is the *answer* to the ethical questions raised by IVF. The problem is more — *how* do we go about exploring these questions?

All would agree that looking at the actual or foreseeable consequences of these new procedures is at least part of the method to be used in exploring these questions. But such a method has very obvious limitations. Judging by consequences needs empirical evidence. Yet empirical evidence is precisely what is not available when one is trying to evaluate new and untried possibilities.

So in one way or another the various lines of argument put forward by the different churches turn once more to the fundamental 'datum' of *human sexuality*. And in looking again at human sexuality, they also take a fresh look at the 'goods' of marriage which have been drawn from the datum of human sexuality.

The God-given link between love and procreation in marriage

As we saw in Chapter 1, the position put forward by the 'majority' of the Catholic Bishops Joint Committee in Bio-Ethical Issues claims that procreation must not be separated from sexual intercourse since that is the God-given locus where the procreational and relational 'goods' are held together essentially. It is there that we touch on something which pertains to the very core of what it means to be human. That is the boundary beyond which we must not go. That is the limit to our dominion over nature. Once that line is crossed, we have left God's meaningful creation behind and we enter into the direction-less wastes of what this position calls human 'unwisdom'. Disaster is inevitable; harmful consequences will follow automatically. It is not surprising that those who hold this position are so emphatic in their rejection of actions which of their very nature thwart this holding together of the procreational and relational 'goods' in the marital act. Because they see things in this light, they truly believe that such actions are trespassing beyond the God-given limits of our dominion over creation and over ourselves as pertaining to the crown of creation.

A very different approach — the one adopted in one form or another by most of the other churches — is to say that it is not possible to isolate any such datum from the field of love and marriage and say that here we touch on the very core of what it means to be human. This approach does not deny the importance of the physical dimension in love and marriage. It recognises that the physical dimension is the necessary medium for interpersonal love — necessary for this love to express itself but also necessary for this love to take shape and be formed in us. Human love goes deeper than physical actions but it needs physical expression if it is to be alive and grow and express itself. The heart of being human lies in the integrity of our relationships. Love, marriage and parenthood are central to this, obviously. According to this approach what lies at the heart of love, marriage and parenthood cannot be fully enshrined within the limits of a physical act, however powerful that action may be as an expression of what love is all about.

In the end, this approach would argue, the heart of love, marriage and parenthood is only revealed through a variety of indications — almost a case of 'by their fruits you shall know them'. That is why this kind of argument from consequences is far from being a full-blown consequentialist argument in its basic inspiration. It takes very seriously the basic question posed earlier: can IVF (either in its simple form without any donor involvement or even with some kind of donor involvement) be a true expression of Christian love? However, it sees no effective way to answer that question other than by examining what will be the consequences flowing from the use of IVF in its different forms. If it can see that IVF will be predominantly harmful to all the persons involved and to the human institution of marriage itself, it will conclude that IVF is not an acceptable way to approach married love and parenthood. It will take this as an indication that IVF is outside the pattern of human loving and parenting designed for us in his wisdom by God. It is obvious that in this approach the argument from consequences relies on some kind of essentialist base. In examining whether IVF causes more 'harm' than 'good', what is considered 'harm' and 'good' is interpreted in the light of what is believed to favour true human living and loving — in other words, what is in accord with the 'good' of marriage, the 'good' of parenthood, the 'good' of children etc.

The deliberately childless marriage — a Christian vocation?

How central are children to marriage is an issue raised in *Choices in Childlessness*. This Report notes that, though the 'childless' marriage is usually seen by Christians (and others) as a misfortune, there are an increasing number of marriages today which are *deliberately* childless. The Report poses the question: is the deliberately childless marriage unchristian (and even inhuman) or does it have a fruitfulness of its own which is distinct from childbearing? It sees this as an important theological question to be faced by the Christian churches today:

> 'The deliberate choice of childlessness, now openly possible through the use of efficient contraception, raises deep theological issues. It certainly calls into question the traditional understanding of marriage. Some Christians have begun to develop a theological framework within which deliberate childlessness within marriage may be embraced as a vocation. Others, however, do not see it as a valid choice if marriage is still to retain its traditional significance and meaning. For virtually the whole of Christian history until now it has been unthinkable for a married couple deliberately to choose not to have children.

Many couples, of course, finding themselves unable to have children of their own, have chosen to remain childless rather than to adopt and foster other's children. They have put their own misfortune to creative use. But misfortune it was, and not a deliberate choice. . . . Because of its radical departure from social expectations and centuries of Christian teaching voluntary childlessness raises new theological and ethical questions.' (p.8)

Choices in Childlessness does more than merely pose this question. It makes an initial and very helpful attempt to give some kind of Christian response to it. It begins by facing a prior question: why do, or should, Christians have children? The Report's answer is both enlightening and inspiring:

'. . . "having children for Christians is a vocation — it is one of the highest callings that we have in such a community" (Hauerwas) . . . in having children Christians are offering a gift and service both to God and to the community.
. . . children are not possessions. They belong to themselves, to the community and to God, and are nobody's possessions. It might be better, from this point of view, not to say that they are given to us, but that they are "entrusted" to us. They belong to God, and he entrusts them to us as potential sons and daughters of his own. They draw forth our love while refusing to be the extension of ourselves. In learning to love our chidren as other than ourselves — they are ours, and yet they are not ours — we learn what is the essential structure of love itself, in which mutual belonging and mutual difference are held together in one spirit. Thus at the same time as loving our children we learn to love our "neighbour" outside our immediate family circle. From a Christian point of view, having and rearing children is itself an expression of faith, hope and love, and to speak of having children in terms of gift is to suggest that in giving us children God also wills to give us himself. In short, a responsible Christian's decision to procreate sets this very decision within the context of God's kingdom of grace, in which he is himself both giver and gift.' (p.30)

Having stressed 'the fundamental importance of children in and for the Christian community' (p.31), *Choices in Childlessness* goes on to examine what it calls a 'vocational liberty of choice'. It states: 'Just as an individual may consider whether he may have a special vocation to celibacy, so too a Christian couple may consider whether they have a special vocation to childlessness.' (p.31) It expands that statement as follows:

'To suggest that there might be a special vocation to marry but to have no children seems to suggest a radical departure from Christian tradition. However, it might be replied that such a suggestion would in fact be a new development of the tradition. It would still be true that children are a gift of God to the Christian community. It would also be true that there would be a general expectation that Christians will marry and have children. This is in the nature of things still likely to be the vocation of the majority. Nevertheless, just as some Christians may find good reasons for proving exceptions to this general expectation by opting for celibacy, so there might be others who would also find good reasons for proving exceptions by opting for marriage but marriage without children. Both those who opt for celibacy and those who opt for marriage without childen would have to assure themselves that they really have good reasons for believing that they have this special vocation. Such reasons should spring from Christian rather than from selfish considerations. But there is more than one way of Christian obedience and discipleship, of creativity and service.' (p.32)

The issue of deliberate childlessness is not faced by any of the other reports from the different churches. Its relevance is obvious since IVF is being developed as a remedy for the 'tragedy' of childlessness. To present a more positive approach to childlessness might help to alter the 'tragic' image of childlessness. The Free Church Federal Council and the British Council of Churches have done a great service in *Choices in Childlessness* by putting this on the theological agenda and by providing a preliminary theological exploration of the issue.

Love is stronger than genes

Some members of the Church of England Working Party which produced *Personal Origins* believe that it is the quality of the relationship which provides the key to all the questions related to IVF. They are not disregarding the welfare of the children. They are simply saying that the couple's loving relationship is the one essential and indispensable element required for the welfare of the children. If the couple's loving relationship is substantially sound, the personal welfare of the children is assured. Whether artificial procedures are used and whether there is any donor involvement are not matters of decisive significance to the welfare of the child as long as the couple's relationship is right. *Personal Origins* voices this view of some of its Working Party thus:

'. . . we judge that, although everyone is fundamentally influenced and limited by his or her genetic endowment, nevertheless the overriding factor is the social context which can assure proper love, respect and care. To this extent the question of genetic origin is not of fundamental moral importance, when compared with the question of how the child will be loved and cared for.' (n.109)

Summing up

All the Christian churches approach the issue of IVF committed to the same basic Christian and human beliefs and values. They want to assess IVF in the light of these beliefs and values. The major point of difference lies in the insistence by the Roman Catholic position that human procreation must not be separated from its God-given setting of marital intercourse since it is there that the inseparability of the procreational and relational 'goods' is located essentially. To violate this inseparability is tantamount to claiming dominion over the meaning of marriage itself. The other churches agree that there is a God-given meaning to marriage. However, while they recognise the importance of the marital act as a unique and powerful expression of inter-personal love, in the end they believe that it is the relationship of love rather than intercourse itself which is the God-given datum enabling us to understand the meaning of marriage. That is why some Christians are beginning to think that it might be possible for couples to live a vocation of truly life-giving and life-sharing love even when they deliberately decide to have no children in their marriage. It also explains why some Christians believe that a sound marriage based on genuine love provides the only truly essential ingredient needed for parenthood. They would maintain that genetic relationship is of secondary importance in comparison to this.

3
What the churches say about
the embryo

How the different Christian churches interpret the status of the embryo plays a significant part in determining their position on IVF. There are various reasons for this. First of all, it would appear that the actual development of IVF has been dependent on the experimental use of human embryos. Secondly, at present IVF involves the discarding of some embryos since there is a better chance of success when only the best embryos are transferred to the mother's uterus. Hence, the disposal of discarded embryos seems to be a normal element in IVF as currently practised. Thirdly, the development of IVF has made it possible to conduct laboratory research on the human embryo in its early stages of development. This research can take the form of observation or experimentation. Some workers in the field claim that such research provides our only hope of understanding and rectifying certain genetic disorders or diseases; others dispute that claim. Whether and in what circumstances such research would be deemed ethically acceptable will depend on how the status of the embryo is interpreted. This is also true of the further question as to whether it would be ethically acceptable to produce embryos specifically for the purpose of research and experimentation.

How the status of the embryo is to be interpreted is not a new question arising for the first time with the advent of IVF. This question has been pondered down through the centuries in connection with the practice of abortion. It has certainly been a question which has loomed large in the thinking of Christians over the years. Before the 1967 Abortion Act became law, there was an upsurge of discussion within the Christian churches over the morality of abortion and so the status of the embryo came in for renewed examination. The massive increase in the number of abortions in this country since 1967 has caused concern within the churches. As a result, the abortion issue and its related question of the status of the embryo has kept reappearing in some form or other on many church agendas. Consequently, when the churches came to look at the ethics of IVF and found that the status of the embryo came up again in this new context, they were not starting from scratch. Their interpretation of the status of the embryo had already been formulated in their ethical examination of abortion. This is why a book which deals with the Christian churches' approach to IVF would be incomplete without a chapter examining how they tackle the status of the embryo in looking at the ethics of abortion. It also explains why, throughout the rest of this book, the issue of abortion keeps reappearing. This is very evident, for instance, in Chapter 5 on the women's perspective and in the Roman Catholic self-critique presented in Chapter 6. However, whenever abortion is considered in this book, the principal focus is not abortion itself but simply the way the different churches interpret the status of the embryo involved in discussing the ethics of abortion.

Abortion and the status of the embryo in Christian tradition

Probably the most thorough piece of original research dealing with abortion and the status of the embryo in Christian tradition is John Connery, *Abortion: The Development of the Roman Catholic Perspective*, (Loyola University Press, Chicago, 1977). Briefer historical treatments are found in John Noonan, *The Morality of Abortion*, (Cambridge, 1970), Daniel Callahan, *Abortion: Law, Choice and Morality*, (London, 1970), Germain Grisez, *Abortion: The Myths, The Realities and The Arguments*, (New York, 1970) and in the entry on Abortion in Warren T Reich (edit.), *Encyclopedia of Bioethics*, (Collier Macmillan, London, 1978), vol I, pp.1-32. For the purposes of this book, a very brief historical outline of abortion in Christian thinking and practice should be sufficient to situate our present-day discussion of the status of the embryo in its context within the life of the church as it has developed down through the centuries.

From the earliest days abortion was condemned by Christians. It was regarded as sinful right from the moment of conception, although the gravity of the sin and the severity of the penalty varied, depending on whether the foetus was 'unformed' or 'formed'. The offence was considered to be 'homicide' only in the latter instance. Originally, the terms 'unformed' and 'formed' referred to the stage of bodily formation — whether it was recognisably 'human' or not. With the development of the theory of progressive ensoulment (first a vegetable soul, then an animal soul, and finally a human soul), which was dependent on the Aristotelian notion of hylemorphism, the foetus was regarded as 'formed' only when it had reached a sufficient stage of development for it to be apt matter for a human soul. Primitive embryology held that this stage was reached after 40 days in the case of a male embryo and after 80 days in the case of a female embryo! The same primitive embryology viewed the male semen as the only real 'life principle'. Hence, 'wasting seed' was considered a sin against life. The woman's contribution was simply to provide the 'nest' for the seed.

This tradition, which viewed abortion as always wrong (but with a graded scale of wrongness depending on 'formation') was carried over by the Reformers in the sixteenth and seventeenth centuries. At that stage in history it was accepted as part of the common Christian tradition. Only in the seventeenth century did the theory of progressive ensoulment come to be questioned. Initially against great opposition, the Belgian physician, Fienus, argued in favour of 'immediate animation' (i.e. the human soul is present right from the moment of conception). Within the Roman Catholic church his view gained a fuller 'official' standing in 1869 when Pius IX followed it in extending the excommunication for abortion.

Whether abortion was permissible to save the life of the mother was an issue that began to be discussed in the fourteenth century, John of Naples being the first to raise it. He argued that such a life-saving abortion might be permissible prior to the foetus being 'formed'. This discussion continued over succeeding centuries. Some moralists went further and argued that abortion might be permissible to save not just the mother's life but also her good name. This view was eventually condemned.

What are the contemporary positions in the different Christian churches on the issue of abortion? The clearest way to proceed in answering that question might be to examine in turn the positions of those Christian churches which have adopted some kind of 'official' stance on abortion.

THE ROMAN CATHOLIC CHURCH

In its section dealing with reverence for the human person the Second Vatican Council states: 'Life must be safeguarded with extreme care from conception; abortion and infanticide are abominable crimes.' (*Gaudium et Spes*, n.51). This teaching, which simply echoes the teaching of successive popes in recent years, is taken up and explained in much greater detail by the Congregation for the Doctrine of the Faith in its *Declaration on Procured Abortion*, (18 November 1984). This document bases its teaching on Scripture and tradition but argues that it also makes sense in the light of human reason. In addition, it faces some objections which are made against this position. The heart of this teaching is found in nn.12-13 of the Vatican Declaration:

'(12) . . . In reality, respect for human life is called for from the time that the process of generation begins. From the time that the ovum is fertilised, a life is begun which is neither that of the father nor of the mother; it is rather the life of a new human being with his own growth. It would never be made human if it were not human already.

(13) This has always been clear, and discussions about the moment of animation have no bearing on it. Modern genetic science offers clear confirmation. It has demonstrated that from the first instant there is established the programme of what this living being will be: a man, this individual man with his characteristic aspects already well determined. Right from fertilisation the adventure of a human life begins, and each of its capacities requires time — a rather lengthy time — to find its place and to be in a position to act. The least that can be said is that present science, in its most evolved state, does not give any substantial support to those who defend abortion. Moreover, it is not up to biological sciences to make a definitive judgment on questions which are properly philosophical and moral, such as the moment when a human person is constituted or the legitimacy of abortion. From a moral point of view this is certain: even if a doubt existed concerning whether the fruit of conception is already a human person, it is objectively a grave sin to dare to risk murder. "The one who will be a man is already one" (Tertullian, Apologeticum, IX, 8).'

This teaching has been voiced in public statements issued by many Roman Catholic hierarchies throughout the world. In January 1980 the Roman Catholic Archbishops of Great Britain took the rather unusual step of issuing a joint statement on abortion (*Abortion and the Right to Live*, CTS, 1980). Although strong in tone, it is a very sensitive statement and tries to situate the issue of abortion in the wider context of respect for the dignity of each human person and basic human rights. The core of its teaching is brought out very clearly in the following passages:

'(4) The Church speaks out against abortion, as it has from the beginning, because it acknowledges the human rights and dignity of all, including the unborn, and is committed to their defence. There is here a crucial point of principle. It has everything to do with the intrinsic value and inalienable rights of each individual. It is a matter of respect for our neighbour . . .

(11) Even before the processes of human reproduction became well understood, Christian teaching always regarded the unborn, at all stages of pregnancy, as possessed of a distinct, new life which no-one could rightly seek to destroy. For many centuries, Christians like others took for granted scientific and philosophical theories which suggested that the newly-conceived human being did not become formed or ensouled until several weeks after conception.

So in those times the ecclesiastical penalties and censures for causing an abortion early in pregnancy were often less severe than those for abortion in later pregnancy. But throughout those centuries, the Church never wavered in its teaching that abortion, at whatever stage of pregnancy, is seriously wrongful. Today the course of human development is much better understood. Modern science enables us to see better than ever before the fundamental significance of the time of conception.

(12) For at the time of conception there comes into existence a new life. There is a union in which a living cell from the father fertilises a living cell from the mother. That union, a transmission of life, is the beginning of new life. Usually this new life is and will always remain a single individual; sometimes, in ways not fully understood, there may then or a few days later be division resulting for example in identical twins. But scientists can tell us that, from the time of conception, the features which distinguish us from each of our parents — the colour of our eyes, our shape of face, and so on — are all laid down in the "genetic code" that comes into existence then. Each such new life is the life not of a potential human being but of a human being with potential. The development of this potential is normally a process of profound continuity. No-one can point to, say the fourth week of that process, or the eighth, the twelfth, the twentieth, the twenty-fourth or twenty-eighth, and say "That is when I began being me". Birth itself is certainly an event in the life-story of each one of us. But for the beginning of that story we must look to the time of our conception.'

Although the Roman Catholic position opts for fertilisation as the key moment and therefore rules out all abortions regardless of the stage of development of the embryo, nevertheless it does not formally teach that there is full human life present from the moment of fertilisation. Even the statement from Vatican II quoted above was worded very carefully. The reason for this, in the words of its drafters, was 'in order not to have to go into the difficult question of the moment at which the soul is infused'. (cf. Bernard Haring, in Vorgrimler (Edit.), *Commentary on the Documents of Vatican II,* vol V, p.243). Likewise, the *Declaration on Procured Abortion* from the Congregation for the Doctrine of the Faith made the same point in a very illuminating footnote —

'This declaration expressly leaves aside the question of the moment when the spiritual soul is infused. There is not a unanimous tradition on this point and authors are as yet in disagreement. For some it dates from the first instant, for others it could not at least precede nidation [implantation]. It is not within the competence of science to decide between these views, because the existence of an immortal soul is not a question in its field. It is a philosophical problem from

which our moral affirmation remains independent for two reasons: (i) suppos-
ing a later animation, there is still nothing less than a human life, preparing for
and calling for a soul in which the nature received from parents is completed; (2)
on the other hand it suffices that this presence of the soul be probable (and one
can never prove the contrary) in order that the taking of life involve accepting
the risk of killing a man, not only waiting for, but already in possession of his
soul.' (footnote, 19)

The Roman Catholic position has opted for the 'safest' interpretation.
As long as we are not 100% certain, it argues, we must play safe and avoid
all risk of directly killing a fully human being. And since it accepts that
100% certainty on this issue is humanly impossible, it regards its position
on abortion as definitive and unchangeable. Any discussion among theologians, it would claim, can at best be purely theoretical. What must be
done in practice is perfectly clear and beyond question: the life of the
embryo must be fully respected from the moment of conception.
Whether this 'safety first' position is really satisfactory will be discussed
later in Chapter 6.

THE CHURCH OF SCOTLAND

At present, it is difficult to know exactly how the General Assembly of the
Church of Scotland interprets the status of the embryo. A report from the
Board of Social Responsibility was formally accepted by the 1985 General
Assembly. This report advocated a position very close to that of the
Roman Catholic Church. It took as its starting-point an earlier General
Assembly statement of 1966: 'We cannot assert too strongly that the in-
violability of the foetus is one of the fundamentals and its right to life must
be strongly defended.' The Board's 1985 report then continued:

'We re-affirm this assertion on several grounds: the biblical teaching, in which
the unborn child is regarded as bearing the divine image; the assertion of the
creed that Jesus Christ was "conceived by the Holy Ghost", God taking man-
hood to himself in utero; the unbroken tradition of the Christian Church,
whereby the first Christians took over the strong Jewish antipathy to abortion;
and the discoveries of modern genetics and embryology, which confirm us in
our belief that the foetus is an independent being, a tiny member of our species.'
(p.283)

In the light of this basic declaration, the Board were extremely critical of
the 1967 Abortion Act and especially of its practical workings. They went
through it clause by clause, pointing out its deficiencies both in principle

and in practice. Their analysis included the following key statement:

> 'From our belief in the sanctity of all human life we are convinced that the inviolability of the foetus can be brought into question only in the case of risk to maternal life and when all alternatives have been exhausted.' (pp.284-285)

This position did not win unqualified approval. According to Boyd, Callaghan and Shotter, the joint authors of *Life before birth,* (SPCK, 1986): 'Almost immediately after the Assembly accepted this (by a narrow majority), however, the Church of Scotland's leading theologians in the field of Christian ethics publicly dissociated themselves from the decision.' (p.104) Obviously, there will be different views as to who merit the description 'the Church of Scotland's leading theologians in the field of Christian ethics'. What cannot be disputed is the fact that the Board's report did not win unanimous support in the General Assembly. Much of the opposition came from those who interpreted it as putting rape victims in a pastorally intolerable position.

There is little doubt that the Church of Scotland's decision at the 1985 General Assembly was considerably influenced by the thinking of Professor Thomas Torrance, the renowned Professor of Christian Dogmatics at Edinburgh University, 1952-1979, and Moderator of the General Assembly 1976-77. His outraged, though carefully reasoned, reaction to the *Warnock Report* is found in his monograph, *Test-tube Babies: Morals — Science — and the Law,* (Scottish Academic Press, Edinburgh, 1984). It is significant that it appeared the year prior to the 1985 General Assembly. He makes it quite clear that he has no doubt that the human embryo has a rightful claim on our full respect from the first moment of its existence:

> 'There is no scientific doubt about the fact that from the moment of conception the human embryo is genetically complete and must be treated as such, as distinctively human, and not just as a mere biochemical episode or as equivalent to the fertilised egg of an animal or a bit of animal tissue. After all if the human embryo were neither human nor alive it would have no place in research on human beings. If the human embryo is genetically complete and distinctively human from the very beginning, then arguments allowing for scientific experiment or genetic manipulation after a certain period, seven, fourteen days or whatever, are scientifically and morally specious. There is also a serious ambiguity about an argument from the premiss that the embryo is "potentially human", for the potentiality concerned is not of becoming something else but of becoming what it essentially is.
>
> No human being, at any stage in his/her existence may be treated in any way that violates his/her distinctively human nature and status or subjects him or

her to being a means to an end. . . The moral status of a human embryo and its moral claim on our behaviour toward it do not diminish the further back we go in the stages of its development, for even in its most minimal state it must never be treated as a means to an end but be respected in itself in its own independent right. Thus it would seem to be morally indefensible when the need to alleviate infertility is given a higher right than that accorded to the gamete or the embryo.' (pp.2-4)

Whether this 'strong' interpretation of the status of the embryo which was enshrined in the 1985 report is still the 'official' position of the Church of Scotland's General Assembly is far from clear. Reversing the previous year's decision, the 1986 Assembly (in Professor Torrance's absence in Geneva) approved a Deliverance which stated:

'(We). . . reaffirm the position held since 1966, that the criteria for abortion should be that the continuance of the pregnancy would involve serious risk to the life or grave injury to the health, whether physical or mental, of the pregnant woman; and instruct the Board to seek a review of the working of the 1967 Abortion Act, with a view to the eradication of any laxity in its interpretation.'

What remains uncertain is whether the Church of Scotland still stands by the 'strong' interpretation of the status of the embryo which was contained in the 1985 report — a report which also claimed to be based on the 1966 proceedings. It is possible that the 1986 General Assembly saw itself as still maintaining that 'strong' interpretation while modifying the rigour of its practical application. However, the matter is further complicated by the fact that the position of the 1966 General Assembly on the status of the embryo is itself far from clear. The authors of *Life before Death* write:

'The Church of England's "degree of agnosticism" (as Dr Habgood called it) on this question was shared by a Report of the Church of Scotland Social and Moral Welfare Board, the conclusions of which were accepted by the Church's 1966 General Assembly: "Traditional attempts to determine some point during pregnancy at which 'human life begins' are inconclusive and are now irrelevant," the Report stated. But the Board, commending the 1965 Anglican Report, also argued that "the inviolability of the foetus is one of the fundamentals and must be defended".' (p.23)

Following the 1986 General Assembly, the Board of Social Responsibility's study group on abortion will continue with fuller research and wider consultation on the issue of abortion, with special reference to the question of the inviolability of the embryo. A full report is to be presented to the 1987 General Assembly. Perhaps a clearer picture of the Church of Scotland's 'official' position on the status of the embryo might emerge after that.

THE CHURCH OF ENGLAND

In 1965 the Church of England Board for Social Responsibility published *Abortion, An Ethical Discussion* as the Anglican contribution to the debate which led to the 1967 Abortion Act. Not all Anglicans would agree with its position but it was welcomed by the Church Assembly in February 1966 'because it stresses the principle of the sanctity of life for mother and foetus.' Notwithstanding criticisms made of it (e.g. Paul Ramsey, 1970, pp.82-86), it remains the main Church of England official statement dealing specifically with abortion. Its basic position on the status of the embryo is very clearly summarised in the following passage:

'The foetus, as potentially a human life, has a significance which must not be overlooked, minimised or denied. Indeed the problem of abortion is precisely the problem of weighing the claims of the mother against the claims of the foetus and vice versa, when they conflict; though it is important that neither be thought of in isolation from the family group of which they are part.

The foetus is not held to derive its significance from a theory that "the soul enters the body" at some point in time; nor must the foetus be thought of and talked about as if it were already a person. In particular, words like "innocent", which are normally matched with other words like "guilty" in a fully-fledged moral discourse, are questionably meaningful when used of the "life" of the foetus. But . . . it still remains true that the foetus has a moral significance insofar as it is potentially a human life and is likely to become a human person in the normal course of events . . .

Our broad conclusion is that in certain circumstances abortion can be justified. This would be when, at the request of the mother and after the kind of consultation which we have envisaged in this report, it could be reasonably established that there was a threat to the mother's life or well-being, and hence inescapably to her health, if she were obliged to carry the child to term and give it birth. And our view is that, in reaching this conclusion, her life and well-being must be seen as integrally connected with the life and well-being of her family . . . In our view such a consultative procedure could cover those cases where justification for abortion would rest upon there being an assessable risk of a defective or deformed child, as well as cases of incest or rape; though the ground of the decision would be the prognosis concerning the mother as affected by the pregnancy; not the possibility of deformity itself, nor simply the fact (if established) of the act of incest or rape.' (pp.61-62)

Some years later, General Synod, sharing 'the widespread anxiety being felt in the country over the working of the Abortion Act 1967', passed resolutions in February 1974, July 1975 and November 1979 in favour of reforming the current law in order to correct the 'manifest abuses' which were taking place under it. When the Roman Catholic Archbishops issued their Joint Statement on Abortion in January 1980 (cf. pp.50-51 above), the Church of England Board for Social Responsibility issued a statement welcoming its publication. While it acknowledged that it is 'not empowered to issue authoritative statements committing members of the Church of England' and also that 'deep differences of judgment concerning abortion exist within the Church of England, as in many other British Churches', the Board felt sufficiently confident to issue a statement which they considered to be 'well-founded in the Christian moral tradition in which we as Anglicans share'. The first section of this statement is worth quoting in its entirety:

> 'First, the central issue. In the light of our conviction that the foetus has a right to live and develop as a member of the human family, we see abortion, the termination of that life by the act of man, as a great moral evil. We do not believe that the right to life, as a right pertaining to persons, admits of no exceptions whatever; but the right of the innocent to life admits surely of few exceptions indeed. Circumstances exist where the character or location of the pregnancy render the foetus a serious threat to the life or health of the mother; in such circumstances (and they are extremely few and well-known) the foetus could be regarded as an 'aggressor' on the mother. The mother would be entitled to seek protection against the threat to her life and health which the foetal life represented. If in those circumstances a choice had to be made between the life of the mother and the continuation of the pregnancy, precedence should be given to the mother's interests; but such a choice would only arise if no less drastic remedy for the ill existed. The undoubted evil of abortion would in this situation represent the lesser of two evils, only resorted to as the appropriate way of caring for the mother if the evil of a significant threat to her life or health cannot otherwise be avoided.
>
> In a society such as ours, however, with advanced facilities for pre-natal diagnosis and care, such situations are today highly exceptional. Women today turn to abortion, or are encouraged to seek abortion, for quite other reasons, reasons which frequently point to seriously unsatisfactory personal or family circumstances but which cannot on that account morally justify the extreme step of abortion.' *(Abortion: a great moral evil)*

In July 1983 General Synod passed a composite resolution whose first three clauses were:

'This Synod:
(a) believes that all human life, including life developing in the womb, is created by God in His own image and is, therefore, to be nurtured, supported and protected;
(b) views with serious concern the number and consequences of abortions performed in the United Kingdom in recent years;
(c) recognises that in situations where the continuance of a pregnancy threatens the life of the mother a termination of pregnancy may be justified and that there must be adequate and safe provision in our society for such situations.'

In 1985 the Church of England Board for Social Responsibility brought out *Personal Origins,* a report which examined the whole area of human fertilisation and embryology. Although it did not concentrate on the issue of abortion, inevitably it was forced to face once again the question of the status of the embryo. It is evident that there was a radical division of opinion within the Working Party. They resist the temptation to resolve this by appending a minority report; nor did they settle for a vague compromise which would do justice to neither view. Instead they did something far more constructive. Since the convictions of those representing both views turned out to be unshakeable, both sides turned their attention to trying to understand how the opposite view could be held with personal integrity and with serious philosophical, theological and scientific grounding. This was no mean task on such an emotive issue. As they said themselves, 'we have come (not without difficulty) to recognise in both these approaches the possibility of a scientifically judicious and theologically responsible set of convictions.' (n.90)

One position maintains that the story of each individual person goes back to fertilisation. This is making the principal focus the 'continuity of the individual subject'. As the Report says in its account of this view, 'behind every presentation of the individual human phenomenon we are accustomed to discern a subject, a "someone" whom we call by a name, who is the bearer of a particular life history.' (n.87) This view gives the embryo inviolable status from the moment of fertilisation. It is, therefore, equivalent to the position of the Roman Catholic church. It is hard to ascertain whether this view is growing in strength within the Church of England. It is certainly being voiced with greater determination and publicity than previously. A recent example of that is the volume of essays edited by J.H. Channer, entitled *Abortion and the Sanctity of Human Life,* (The Paternoster Press, Exeter, 1985). In his foreward E.L. Mascall writes: 'The primary purpose of this volume . . . is to maintain that, whatever its advantages, real or apparent may be, abortion is immoral because it is the deliberate killing of an innocent and helpless human being; it is an attempt to solve human problems by the short cut of eliminating human beings.' (p.9)

The second position focuses on the phenomenon of consciousness as being the distinctive feature of the human person. This is not demanding that the actual exercise of consciousness be present but it is looking for the minimum condition required for judging when there exists 'a subject capable in principle and in normal cases of exercising some rational or moral capacities.' (n.89) It explains its position as follows:

> 'Adopting the principle that one should err on the side of caution, one may seek to locate the earliest roots of rational, moral and religious activity. One may then look to the first moments of the conscious experience which goes to constitute the basis of later rational thought . . . Such a consciousness, at least in its human form, is causally dependent upon certain physical states, and in particular upon certain structures of the central nervous system and the brain stem. The human subject of consciousness, then, cannot come to exist before the development of a body of a certain degree of complexity. It seems plausible to conclude, argue those who adopt this approach, that the human subject — in the strong sense of "human" in which we recognise humanity as making a special moral claim upon us — cannot take form in an embryonic body which has not yet reached the appropriate stage of differentiation and development.' (n.89)

It will be noticed that this statement expresses in non-technical language a position which is virtually the same as those (mainly Roman Catholics) who are seeking to reinstate, with due allowance for the findings of modern embryology, the early Christian belief in ensoulment only at a stage when the appropriate biological substratum has developed which is capable of sustaining a human soul. The phrase 'human subject of consciousness' could probably be interchanged for 'soul' without any substantial alteration of meaning.

What is particularly illuminating in this Report is the Working Party's attempt to discern their underlying agreement about certain basic principles governing the way they must approach this issue. Because they agree that these basic principles must be respected, they are able to conduct a joint exploration into the scientific, philosophical and Christian respectability of their different positions; and they are able to do this without the two views feeling compelled to take up battle positions against each other. It is a helpful case-study in what might be called 'ecumenism in ethics'!

They agree on four basic principles:

(1) Scientific evidence must be faced honestly, but its significance can only be arrived at by a process of interpretation. The Report states:

'Science, as such, can only report what happens; it cannot interpret it. It cannot tell us whether the genetic structures of individuality are *more important* to our understanding of what it is to be human than (say) the complexification of the nervous system, or vice-versa. A decision between the approaches can only be made on theological or philosophical grounds.' (n.91)

That this principle is also shared by the Roman Catholic position is evident from the 1974 Vatican Declaration on Procured Abortion quoted earlier in this chapter. 'It is not up to biological sciences to make a definitive judgement on questions which are properly philosophical and moral, such as the moment when a human person is constituted . . .' (n.13)

(2) Since the interpretation involved is theological, an examination has to be made as to what light the Bible throws on the issue.

(3) Christian tradition has also to be taken seriously. An interpretation is not truly Christian if it shows no respect for the thinking and beliefs of Christians of earlier ages. On the issue under consideration two complementary strands in Christian tradition are noted: (i) 'Christian thinkers of the past believed both in a decisive moment of beginning, given by a new creative act of God himself, and in the possibility, at least, that such a moment belonged not at the very start of the embryo's physicial development but some way into it.' (n.94); (ii) the practical protection of the early embryo, partially as a safety measure due to uncertainty about the time of animation.

(4) The human status of the embryo is not something dependent on human decision.

'The human status of the unborn child is something which must be discerned, quite apart from our wishes or our decisions, as a reality which simply commands our recognition as of right . . . Some of our contemporaries have hoped to avoid the question of the embryo's status altogether, and have thought it possible to move directly to a purely deliberative question: how are we to act towards the early embryo? The implication of this manoeuvre would seem to be that human status is not so much discerned as conferred.' (n.97)

In June 1985 General Synod, by 150 votes to 127, commended *Personal Origins* 'to the dioceses and to the wider Church for study, debate and response . . .'.

THE METHODIST CHURCH

The Methodist Conference adopted a formal statement on abortion in 1976. The following year the Division of Social Responsibility of the Methodist Church produced a report giving the background to this statement and providing a commentary on it — John Atkinson (edit.), *Abortion reconsidered: The Methodist Statement and its Background,* (Methodist Publishing House, 1977). This report was the fruit of a Methodist revision and reworking of an earlier report which had been prepared by a joint Methodist-Church of England working party. That earlier report had not been accepted for publication by the Church of England Board for Social Responsibility.

The Methodist Conference statement laid out the theological principles on which it based its judgement about abortion.

'(3) The Christian believes that man is a creature of God, made in the divine image, and that human life, though marred, has eternal as well as physical and material dimensions. All human life should therefore be reverenced. The foetus is undoubtedly part of the continuum of human existence, but the Christian will wish to study further the extent to which a foetus is a person. Man is made for relationships, being called to respond to God and to enter into a living relationship with Him. Commanded to love their neighbours, Christians must reflect in human relationships their response to God's love. Although the foetus possesses a degree of individual identity, it lacks independence and the ability to respond to relationships. All *persons* are always our 'neighbours'; other beings may call forth our loving care. In considering the matter of abortion, therefore, the Christian asks what persons, or beings who are properly to be treated wholly or in part as persons, are involved and how they will be affected by a decision to permit or forbid abortion.'

The statement goes on to remind Christians of their duty to stand by people in times of crisis and help them make responsible decisions. It also warns that human judgements may be impaired by sin and that abortion decisions may be made 'in a context of selfishness, carelessness or exploitation'. (n.5) It then proceeds to analyse the issues involved:

'(6) On one side of the abortion debate is the view which seeks to uphold the value and importance of all forms of human life by asserting that the foetus has an inviolable right to life and that there must be no external interference with the process which will lead to the birth of a living human being. The other side of the debate emphasises the interests of the mother. The foetus is totally dependent on her for at least the first twenty weeks of the pregnancy and, it is therefore argued, she has a total right to decide whether or not to continue the pregnancy. It is further argued that a child has the right to be born healthy and wanted.

(7) Both views make points of real value. On the one hand, the significance of human life must not be diminished; on the other hand, abortion is unique because of the total physical dependence of the foetus on the mother, to whose life, capacities or existing responsibilities the foetus may pose a threat of which she is acutely aware. It is necessary both to face this stark conflict of interests and to acknowledge that others are also involved — the father, the existing children of the family, the extended family, and society generally.

(8) From the time of fertilisation, the foetus is a separate organism, biologically identifiable as belonging to the human race and containing all the genetic information. It will naturally develop into a new living human individual. A few days after fertilisation, implantation (or nidation) takes place; it is significant that in the period before nidation a very large number of fertilised ova perish. At some time after the third month, the 'quickening' occurs — an event which is of significant, perhaps crucial, moment for the mother. Not earlier than the 20th week, the foetus becomes viable, i.e. able to survive outside the womb if brought to birth.

(9) There is never any moment from conception onwards when the foetus totally lacks human significance — a fact which may be overlooked in the pressure for abortion on demand. However the degree of this significance manifestly increases. At the very least this suggests that no pregnancy should be aborted after the point when the aborted foetus would be viable. . . .'

The Methodist position, therefore, insists on respect for the embryo but it maintains that this respect should be in keeping with the embryo's developing human status. It sees the achievement of the human dignity of the embryo as a gradual process and does not identify any one stage of the process as completely determinative.

THE BAPTIST UNION OF GREAT BRITAIN AND IRELAND

Although the Baptist Union of Great Britain and Ireland is merely a voluntary association of some 2,400 local Baptist churches, some indication of Baptist thinking can be drawn from the evidence they submitted to the Warnock Committee. This document opens with a very closely reasoned analysis of how Christian moral judgements are made. Because this lays the basis for the position they adopt with regard to abortion, it is worth quoting at length from this section of their evidence:

'1 . . . there are no fixed and universal moral rules available which might be simply applied to a situation. Rather, Christian ethics must seek to find the demand with which God confronts us in any particular situation. While God has a will for man's life, any set of rules could only be a relative and approximate reflection of this will. God's demand is a call for love (which includes justice) and is expressed in compassion in a particular situation, and thus the details of the situation itself must be examined to discover its reality and through this the moral demand.

However, in coming to a decision as to what is the loving thing to do, there are also certain "claims" which pre-exist any particular situation. These are not fixed rules, but obligations which have the right to first consideration. They demand a bias in their favour. The strength of these prior "claims" is such that, though they can be set aside, they would have to be clearly outweighed by any contrary factors in the situation itself, and the balance of doubt would always lie on their side.

Such prior "claims" include:

(1) natural rights;

(2) promises already made or covenants entered into;

(3) "the form of the Christ in the here and now" — viz. the way in which the Christian community perceives life as being shaped in the present by the image of the true humanity in Christ. This Christian life-style emerges through the common mind of the Church today, and draws upon the heritage of Christian tradition, particularly biblical principles which embody the experience of the past community of faith.

2. This kind of ethic, which recognises that there are intrinsic goods (God's will for mankind) and, conversely, evils but that no human expression of these can ever be absolute, has a further important consequence for moral decisions; it confirms the notion of "the lesser of two evils" in some situations. To refuse to recognise this is to blunt moral sensitivity. Situations are morally complex, and to recognise that an action includes an evil element but is the right one to take nevertheless in a particular situation, will keep us from being hardened to that action, which in other situations might be both evil and wrong. Responsibility may thus inevitably involve a sense of guilt, though the guilt does not necessarily fall upon the persons directly involved. This has obvious relevance for the present questions which may require the taking of the life of an embryo . . .'
(p.2)

The Evidence then proceeds to identify empirical factors in a situation which would help to shape moral judgement. It then goes on to identify the 'claims' or over-riding obligations which it has referred to in the above quotation. It presents these claims under two headings, the first being 'the obligation to preserve and fulfil human life'. It immediately makes a point which has been strongly emphasised by some of the other Christian churches — the source of the value of human life is not any human judgement but God himself. 'The claim to preserve life does not rest simply upon any human judgement about the intrinsic value of life. Belief in God as "Other" than man as Lord of life and death means that there is a transcendent claim upon man which safeguards one human being from being manipulated by another.' (p.4) It expands this 'claim' in terms of the healing and enrichment of life, not just its preservation. And since the value of human life has its ultimate basis in God himself, the Evidence rejects any attempt to make value dependent upon comparative assessments of quality. 'Any attempt by man himself to decide that a certain kind of life has more or less value than another is self-justification which denies man's creaturely status.' (p.4) That is why it challenges any assumption that the discovery of a genetic defect in an embryo is sufficient grounds for an abortion — 'it is not self-evident that such a life is valueless or without meaning'. (p.4)

The question of the status of the embryo is discussed under the heading of the second 'claim' which is described as 'the obligation not to reduce man's humanity'. As will be seen later, the Evidence prefers to use the term 'personality' in place of 'humanity'. It insists that a human being is more than a physical entity, though 'Christian theology at present rarely defines this "more" in terms of a separate and separable component such as "an immortal soul".' (p.5) While acknowledging his creaturely limitations, it stresses a human being's 'freedom to transcend himself and his environment (for example, in his awareness of being conscious).' It comes to the conclusion: 'although this "more" in man is finally elusive, it has to do with his being called to live in a personal and responsible relationship with God.' (p.5)

Using the expression 'human personality' to mean something like 'full humanity' or 'human being in the full sense of the word', the Evidence faces the question: 'when can human personality, as distinct from life only, be said to begin'. It looks at four possible moments — (1) fertilisation; (2) implantation; (3) 'quickening'; (4) birth. It then continues:

> 'It is easy, in our opinion, to dismiss (3) and (4) on scientific and medical evidence. There is no doubt that life begins before birth, and also before the first movements are felt.
>
> To answer the case for (1) and (2) is more difficult. After fertilisation, the embryo has the potential to develop into a human being, but until implantation this potential cannot be realised. Life depends on a positive interaction with the environment for its sustenance and until implantation there is no such interaction. The bundle of cells that make up the embryo has only a small internal sup-

ply of food which is quickly used up and, if no implantation occurs, pregnancy will not take place. This bundle of cells is not dead, but it is not a human personality. Just as the sperm or the ovum are alive but have no ability to keep living and growing, so the embryo is alive but will not keep living and growing until it is implanted into the wall of the uterus. Until a foetus is viable outside the womb it can only be a *potential* human personality, but it nevertheless deserves respect on precisely that account. Thus the question as to when personality begins cannot be answered absolutely, since man is a psychosomatic unity. But there is clearly an increasing weight of claim to respect as a "potential personality", as the embryo increases in that potential. At *all* stages there is a need for social awareness of respect for potential personality (to whom, the Christian adds, God relates Himself in covenant love); but decisions about genetic engineering or manipulating of germ-line cells and embryos must take into account the point of development. With increasing growth of an embryo the greater would need to be the weight of argument for altering or terminating that potential personality.' (p.6)

In their later Response to the *Warnock Report*, the Baptist Union of Great Britain give a fairly strong welcome to the Report. They note that it accords with their own submission in arguing that 'the development of personhood is a complex matter, and that no clear boundary can be drawn as to when personhood begins.' (Response, p.3) They also welcome the Report's view that 'the embryo deserves respect on that account at all stages of its growth, even though it cannot be regarded as having exactly the same status as a human person who has been born.' (p.3) and they agree with the Report that 'the embryo cannot be simply defined as "a human person" and that the respect accorded to it cannot be absolute.' (p.3) However, they are unhappy with the Report to the extent that it seems to offer no positive description of the status of the embryo equivalent to the 'potential personality' put forward by themselves in their Evidence. Nevertheless, they admit that Expression of Dissent B embraces their view 'unambiguously' in ascribing to the embryo 'potential for becoming a human person'. They view this lack of positive description as a crucial omission since making moral judgements involves weighing 're-spect for the embryo against the needs of living persons'. This leads them to insist:

'The "claim" of the embryo upon our respect ought to have the full weight of potential personhood as given by God, and recognising this unambiguously might well lead to some slightly different conclusions from the Report.' (Response, p.3)

Summing up

For all practical purposes the position of the Roman Catholic Church equates the status of the embryo with the status of any other living human being and determines its dignity accordingly. Insofar as IVF, at least as currently practised, seems to necessitate the production of surplus embryos, it stands condemned by the Roman Catholic position. Even prescinding from whether these surplus embryos are allowed to die or are used for experimental purposes, it is offensive to their human dignity deliberately to produce them as surplus in the first instance without their being given any chance to develop naturally. This is the basic objection to IVF which is made by the Catholic Bishops' Joint Committee on Bio-Ethical Issues (cf. nn.7-15). In contrast to their line of argument examined in Chapter 1, the Committee were unanimous in voicing this objection and were even prepared to state that 'certain aspects of much current IVF practice are fundamentally unacceptable and ought to be prohibited by any civilized community'. (n.11)

Some individual members of the other Christian churches share this view. This is particularly true of the Church of Scotland whose General Assembly formally accepted this position in 1985, even though they modified it the following year.

The Methodist Conference Statement on Abortion (1976) opts for a developing human status for the embryo or foetus. Although each Baptist Church is free to adopt its own position, the Baptist Union seems to favour a similar position, as does the Church in Wales and the Free Churches. This means that they would not view causing the death of the early foetus as taking human life in the proper sense of the word. In practice, therefore, they too would have no objection, at least on this score, to IVF as currently practised and likewise they would accept the death of surplus embryos provided this was a necessary accompaniment to a responsible IVF programme. They would also accept experimentation on surplus embryos for substantial human health benefits. They would not limit this experimentation to the first 14 days but they would demand an increasingly graver justifying reason in proportion to the more developed stage of the embryo or foetus.

The above summary limits itself to the differing views of the churches on the status of the embryo. As has been seen in Chapter 1, many of the churches object to IVF, or at least have reservations about certain aspects of it, on grounds other than the status of the embryo.

4

Analysing what the churches say about the embryo

What conclusions are we to draw from the previous chapter? Are the Christian churches so hopelessly divided about the kind of reverence due to the embryo that any kind of agreed position is totally impossible? I would suggest that that is far from being the case.

On the abortion issue itself there is wide agreement on certain basic principles. That in itself should be sufficient to enable constructive inter-church dialogue to take place. Nevertheless, it cannot be denied that, at a practical level especially, there are one or two very fundamental points of disagreement between some of the churches. These disagreements have to be acknowledged and listened to respectfully, if any inter-church dialogue on this issue is to be anything more than an empty gesture of ecumenical politeness. Dialogue over our disagreements can only be constructive if churches enter into it in a spirit of mutual sharing and openness. That means that churches will want to share the truth as far as they see it; but also, as far as possible, they will want to receive from each other a deeper understanding of that truth. That might well involve the painful process of listening to and trying to appreciate the reasons why some other Christian churches cannot share some of the beliefs they feel most deeply about on this issue. Dialogue conducted in such a spirit will not be aimed at trying to 'win over' other churches to one's own point of view. Instead it will be based on a deep desire that God's Spirit will win over all the churches to a deeper and more widely shared understanding of the truth.

There is almost complete unanimity among the churches regarding the way Christians should approach the question of the status of the embryo.

A context of respect: God is the ultimate source of human dignity

All the Christian churches agree that the most fundamental context for discussing the status of the embryo is that of *respect* for the God-given dignity of human beings. For Christians the ultimate source of this dignity lies in the fact that human beings are made in the image of God and are called into intimate relationship with God in and through Jesus Christ. However they interpret the status of the embryo, all the churches situate the discussion in this overall context. As shall be seen later, this has important implications for the possibility of inter-church dialogue.

THE CHURCH OF SCOTLAND

'The Christian perspective starts from the position that human beings have been created by God and are loved by God. Made "in the image of God and after his likeness", man is unique and has been endowed with faculties which enable him to enter into a personal relationship with his creator, and undertake responsibility for the creation on behalf of and alongside his creator. However, it is not just to the creative activity of God we must look, but to the Incarnation and to his saving activity. God in Christ underlines not only the uniqueness of man, but the attitude of God, which is that His love does not depend on our achievements or abilities. The value of human life and the dignity of life, derive from how God regards and treats us, and not on any status which legal or moral codes and conventions may confer at particular ages and stages of development. Thus, human beings may never treat each other as means to ends, but only as ends, and as ends backed by ultimate sanction of God's own being and love incarnate in Jesus Christ. No human being at any stage in his or her development may be treated in a way that violates his/her distinctively human nature and status, or subjects him/her to being a means to an end, even where that end is the greater health and happiness of other beings.' (p.288)

METHODISM

'The Christian believes that man is a creature of God, made in the divine image, and that human life, though marred, has eternal as well as physical and material dimensions. All human life should therefore be reverenced. The foetus is undoubtedly part of the continuum of human existence, but the Christian will wish to study further the extent to which a foetus is a person. Man is made for relationships, being called to respond to God and to enter into a living relationship with Him. Commanded to love their neighbours, Christians must reflect in human relationships their response to God's love. Although the foetus possesses a degree of individual identity, it lacks independence and the ability to respond to relationships. All *persons* are always our 'neighbours'; other beings may call forth our loving care. In considering the matter of abortion, therefore, the Christian asks what persons, or beings who are properly to be treated wholly or in part as persons, are involved and how they will be affected by a decision to permit or forbid abortion.' (n.3)

THE BAPTIST UNION OF GREAT BRITAIN AND IRELAND

'. . . the claim to preserve life does not rest simply upon any human judgement about the intrinsic value of life. Belief in God as "Other" than man as Lord of life and death means that there is a transcendent claim upon man which safeguards one human being from being manipulated by another . . . Belief in God as Redeemer of life means that Christian concern is not only for the preservation of life, but also for its healing and enrichment. Christian faith has a dynamic concept of the personality as being in the process of growth, in a relationship of love with a God who enters into covenant with man. This includes the calling of man to a work of co-creativity with God in making life whole . . . God Himself as Creator and Redeemer gives value to human life. So any attempt by man himself to decide that a certain kind of life has more or less value than another is self-justification which denies man's creaturely status. . . Made in the image of God, man has a certain freedom to transcend himself and his environment. . ., though as a creature he is also limited. Thus, although this "more" in man is finally elusive, it has to do with his being called to live in personal and responsible relationship with God.' (*Submission to Warnock Committee,* pp.4-5)

THE FREE CHURCH FEDERAL COUNCIL AND THE BCC

'. . . human beings have a value more fundamental than that which any human society may ascribe to them. They are made in the image of God, redeemed by the sacrifice of Christ and called to an eternal destiny. Thus it is God who has given them their essential humanity, both in relation to himself and in relation to one another. They have a value in his sight not because of their own achievements or deserts, but because they are the recipients of his creative and redemptive love.' (p.24)

ROMAN CATHOLIC CHURCH

'God, who has fatherly concern for everyone, has willed that all men should constitute one family and treat one another in a spirit of brotherhood. For having been created in the image of God, who "from one man has created the whole human race and made them live all over the face of the earth" (Acts 17,26), all men are called to one and the same goal, namely, God Himself . . . Coming down to practical and particularly urgent consequences, this Council lays stress on reverence for man: everyone must consider his every neighbour without exception as another self. . . Furthermore, whatever is opposed to life itself, such as any type of murder, genocide, abortion . . . these things and others of their like are infamies indeed . . . they are a supreme dishonour to the Creator.' (*Gaudium et Spes,* nn.24 & 27)

CHURCH OF ENGLAND

'According to Christian tradition, human beings are made in the image of God (Gen. l.26). This bestows upon them a unique status in creation. "Thou hast made him little less than a god crowning him with glory and honour" (Psalm 8.5). At different times of the Church's tradition, various aspects of this 'image' have been emphasised. For some it resides principally in our capacity for relationship with God and with our fellow human beings. For others it lies in the human capacity for reason and for exercising responsibility. For yet others it lies in man's capacity to have dominion over the world and to use this power responsibly. These capabilities are inherent in humanity and raise human beings to the special dignity of persons. . .

(2.3) Because human beings are made in the image of God, to treat them not as persons to be respected but as things which may be manipulated is to violate their God-given nature. Although in few Christian traditions is human life absolutely sacrosanct, it is always worthy of very high respect and of special protection from the law.' (*Human Fertilisation and Embryology: Board for Social Responsibility Response to the Warnock Report*, nn.2.l & 2.3)

As well as placing the debate firmly in the context of respect for the Godgiven dignity of human beings, some of the above texts go further and affirm this respect, regardless of whether the embryo is to be considered a human person or not. Though it is not clear what precisely is meant by this respect, it is quite clear that it is understood to have some very positive content.

Respect involves the recognition of dignity, not the conferral of dignity

The Christian churches agree that this respect is not something that we are free to give or withhold. It is something demanded of us. *Reverence* might be a more appropriate word than respect. Reverence is not an attitude which one adopts by free choice. It is the natural reaction of any human being as he or she stands before the mystery of human life; and I use the word "mystery" in its deepest sense to denote a level of reality which is so rich in meaning that, though we can glimpse it partially, we can never fully comprehend it. Consequently, all the churches insist that human dignity is not something "conferred" by society. It is something which is simply "recognised" with reverence.

ROMAN CATHOLIC CHURCH

'The first right of the human person is his life. He has other goods and some are more precious, but this one is fundamental — the condition of all the others. It does not belong to society, nor does it belong to public authority in any form to recognise this right for some and not for others; all discrimination is evil, whether it be founded on race, sex, colour or religion. It is not recognition by another that constitutes this right. This right is antecedent to its recognition; it demands recognition and it is strictly unjust to refuse it.' (*Declaration on Procured Abortion*, n.11)

THE CHURCH OF ENGLAND

'The human status of the unborn child is something which must be discerned, quite apart from our wishes or our decisions, as a reality which simply commands our recognition as of right . . . Some of our contemporaries have hoped to avoid the question of the embryo's status altogether, and have thought it possible to move directly to a purely deliberative question: how are we to act towards the early embryo? The implication of this manoeuvre would seem to be that human status is not so much discerned as conferred.' (*Personal Origins*, n.97)

THE BAPTIST UNION OF GREAT BRITAIN AND IRELAND

'. . . the claim to preserve life does not rest simply upon any human judgment about the intrinsic value of life. Belief in God as "Other" than man as Lord of life and death means that there is a transcendent claim upon man which safeguards one human being from being manipulated by another . . . God Himself as Creator and Redeemer gives value to human life. So any attempt by man himself to decide that a certain kind of life has more or less value than another is self-justification which denies man's creaturely status.' (*Submission to the Warnock Committee*, p.4)

THE FREE CHURCH FEDERAL COUNCIL AND THE BBC

'Human beings have a value more fundamental than that which any human society may ascribe to them. They are made in the image of God, redeemed by the sacrifice of Christ and called to an eternal destiny. Thus it is God who has given them their essential humanity, both in relation to himself and in relation to one another. They have a value in his sight not because of their own achievements or deserts, but because they are the recipients of his creative and redemptive love.' (*Choices in Childlessness*, p.24)

THE CHURCH OF SCOTLAND

'Human life is intrinsically meaningful: it is to be understood in terms of the will and purpose of God involving mutual obligation within society.' (p.289)

The churches thus agree that they are committed to respect for human life and for the life of every human being and that this commitment is not dependent on their own free choice. It is a commitment that flows naturally from their recognition of humankind's creaturely status. It pertains to their attitude of reverence before God and before the wonder of his creation which find its crown in humanity itself and most especially in Jesus through whom humanity becomes the expression of God's own love.

Discerning the respect owed to the human embryo

It is from this shared belief that the different Christian churches approach the question: what about the embryo? Faced with the human embryo are they in the presence of a being which demands from them exactly the same reverence as is due to every other human being? What is the status of the human embryo?

Although this is a question of special concern to Christians, it is a question to be faced by every person who takes life seriously and who is committed to the basic value of respect for human dignity. Answering this question is, therefore, a shared endeavour. The churches have no hot-line to heaven, giving them a pre-packaged answer to this question. The churches have to join the rest of humanity in their endeavour to answer this question satisfactorily. That is why one essential element in the Christian approach must be to *listen* attentively.

LISTENING TO THE SCIENTIFIC AND EMPIRICAL EVIDENCE

The churches must listen to the scientific and empirical evidence. What do the human sciences tell us about the human embryo? In their reports all the churches have taken very seriously this 'listening' part of their role. They all describe what they have heard the geneticist and embryologists saying to them. Briefly, they have heard them saying: (1) the embryo is human; it belongs to the human species. (2) it is genetically complete. (3) barring accidents and given the right environment, it will naturally and from its own inner dynamism develop into what everyone would acknowledge to be a human being in the proper sense of the term. This is the scientific evidence and none of the churches would dispute it. Some people would also consider the two phenomena of twinning and foetal wastage to be relevant empirical evidence. (cf. Chapter 6)

INTERPRETING THE EVIDENCE

Empirical evidence needs to be 'interpreted'. To discern whether or not this evidence forces us to the interpretation that the human foetus is a human being in the proper sense of that term is outside the domain of the scientists. That is a question for the philosopher or the theologian. This point is made very explicitly by some of the churches and none of the churches seem to deny it in any way:

> 'Science, as such, can only report what happens; it cannot interpret it. It cannot tell us whether the genetic structures of individuality are *more important* to our understanding of what it is to be human than (say) the complexification of the nervous system, or *vice versa*. A decision between the approaches can only be made on theological or philosophical grounds.' (*Personal Origins*, n.91)

> 'It is not up to biological sciences to make a definitive judgment on questions which are properly philosophical and moral, such as the moment when a human person is constituted or the legitimacy of abortion . . . (The) question of when the spiritual soul is infused . . . is not within the competence of science . . . It is a philosophical problem . . .' (*Declaration on Procured Abortion*, n.13 and footnote 19)

> 'Science and technology cannot provide the answers to the deepest and far-reaching questions about the purpose and meaning of human life. That is not their function.' (*Choices in Childlessness*, p.36)

THE CHRISTIAN CONTRIBUTION TO THIS INTERPRETATION

It is obvious that the churches are claiming that it is precisely in this area of *interpreting* the empirical evidence that they have something specific to contribute. Yet it should be noted that by stating that this question is 'philosophical', they are thereby admitting that the right to speak on this issue is not reserved to the churches. Philosophers (those who ponder deeply on the meaning of life) also have to be listened to seriously on this issue.

What is the specific contribution that the Christian churches have to make? It is not simply their reverence for God's creation and their commitment to respect for human dignity. Many men and women who are not Christians have a very profound reverence for life and deeply respect human dignity. It is more the fact that they have an even richer motivation for this reverence and respect. Their Christian faith enables them to see further beneath the surface of life. The creation they reverence is not just an object of natural wonder; it is the creation which has at its heart Jesus Christ, the Word of God made flesh. And the human being whose dignity they respect is not just the master-piece of God's creative genius; through the Incarnation each and every human being is called to be a member of God's own family.

This privileged vision of the Christian churches does not provide an immediate answer to the question about the status of the human embryo. However, it does provide a number of reasons why the Christian contribution can lay claim to a special hearing:

(1) The Christian churches can see that this question has an even greater importance than might first meet the eye. Its implications go far deeper than one might imagine. They should, therefore, have a greater sense of urgency in trying to resolve this question.

(2) The Christian churches' awareness of sin makes them more alert to the possibility that the answer to the question regarding the status of the embryo might be unduly influenced by a number of factors which do not relate directly to the status of the embryo itself. Such factors could be to do with the more immediate happiness and needs of the people involved; pressures created by the alleged advantages of embryo experimentation; the need for security felt by individuals or even by some churches or church institutions and how this can be perceived to be threatened by the questioning of clear, firm teaching; personal experiences causing one to have greater concern for either the embryo or for the mother and her family; approaches to motherhood and family which portray abortion either as a symbol of a woman's freedom or as a threat to her security (cf. Chapter 5), etc.

(3) The Christian vision has meant that down through the ages the Christian church or churches have been deeply involved in life and death issues and many Christians have devoted their lives to promoting deeper respect for men and women who have been cast aside by society at large. Although their record on this matter is very far from being unblemished, the Christian churches' commitment has been sufficiently consistent to justify claiming that they have an 'instinct' for what is right and wrong in matters involving respect or disrespect for the human person. To identify this 'instinct' with the action of the Holy Spirit would be to over-state the churches' claim. The action of the Holy Spirit is not enclosed within the confines of the churches; and the churches are affected by many other influences besides the Holy Spirit. Nevertheless, when this instinct is true, the churches would

interpret it as the action of the Spirit. That is why the churches would all agree that, like any other issue, this question cannot be considered properly by Christians in isolation from the Spirit-inspired Christian scriptures and Christian tradition down through the centuries.

So the Christian churches bring *a more profound sense of reverence* to the common human search to discern the true human significance of the human embryo. That is why all the churches, without exception as far as I know, would say very strongly that *reverence and respect is owed to the human embryo from the moment of conception*. This is because they all recognise that (i) the human embryo is human; (ii) it is human life; (iii) it is a necessary stage of human development; and (iv) there is a true continuity between this embryo and the human person it will develop into. There is complete agreement on all that.

What this reverence means in terms of practical behaviour needs to be unpacked by the churches. At the very least, all would say that it means that the human embryo cannot be treated as just a blob of tissue. As we have seen, the churches agree that their sense of reverence and respect recognises that the human embryo has a certain intrinsic 'value'. This means that its good (its life, growth and development) must be respected and can only be put in second place or even sacrificed if it is in direct conflict with some higher good related to the dignity of human beings.

DIFFERENT CHRISTIAN INTERPRETATIONS — RESOLVING CONFLICT SITUATIONS

It is precisely at this point that there is a dividing of the ways between the Christian churches. All would agree that the human embryo has 'value' and must be given respect. The disagreement concerns what precisely is the 'value' of the human embryo. One view, represented most clearly by the Roman Catholic church and the Church of Scotland 1985 General Assembly, states that it has exactly the same value as any other human being. Another view, represented by a strong body of opinion in the Church of England, states that its value, prior to the stage of definitive individuation, is less than that of a human being in the proper sense of the word. A third view, represented by the Methodist Conference, would say that its value depends on its stage of development. It has the progressively increasing value of, say, a not-yet implanted eight-cell embryo, a two-, five- or eight-month old foetus.

Since all these different interpretations start from an attitude of reverence for human dignity, they all bring this reverence to bear on resolving the dilemmas which arise when there is a conflict of values. Obviously, however, there will be a different end-result depending on the value given to the embryo.

When the value given to the embryo is exactly the same as that given to any other human being, reverence will demand that the good of the embryo is not directly sacrificed for the good of any of the human beings involved. According to this view, therefore, reverence for human dignity would rule out every form of direct abortion and it would also exclude any use of embryos for experimental purposes.

When full human value is given to the embryo only after the point of definitive individuation has been reached, then prior to that moment the good of the embryo will take second place when it is in conflict with the good of human beings to whom full reverence is owed. According to this view, therefore, reverence for human dignity would justify experimentation on the early embryo if it is judged that the results of such experimentation are likely to bring substantial human benefits, thus enabling other human beings to live their lives more in keeping with human dignity.

When the human embryo is considered to have a less-than-fully-human but progressively increasing value up to the time of birth, then reverence for human dignity would justify not only experimentation on embryos for serious human purposes but also abortion right through the whole of pregnancy. It would be a violation of human dignity, according to this view, to subordinate the good of a human being to whom full reverence is owed to that of a being to which, despite its intrinsic value, less than full reverence is due. However, the reasons for abortion would need to increase in their gravity in proportion to the lateness of the pregnancy.

Why the churches differ in their interpretation — the significance of potential

Why is it that there is a divergence of view among the Christian churches regarding the status of the embryo? After all, they are faced with exactly the same genetic and embryological evidence. It is not the evidence they differ on; it is how this evidence is to be interpreted. Yet interpretation is not a matter of purely arbitrary, personal whim. Interpretation means applying certain criteria to the evidence in order to determine its real significance. Therefore, if the churches differ in their interpretation, it must be because the criteria they are applying are different.

The criteria we apply in our process of interpretation are drawn from our way of seeing things. And our way of seeing things simply means 'our philosophy of life'. If the criteria applied by the churches are different, it may well be due to some 'philosophical' difference between the churches. One such philosophical difference is clearly situated in their approach to and understanding of *potency* and *act*. Some contrasting statements from the various churches will illustrate this point very vividly:

THE ROMAN CATHOLIC CHURCH

'It (the fertilised ovum) would never be made human if it were not human already . . . "The one who will be a man is already one" (Tertullian, *Apologeticum*, X, 8).' (*Declaration on Procured Abortion*, nn.12 & 13)

'Each such new life is the life not of a potential human being but of a human being with potential.' (Joint Statement of the Roman Catholic Archbishops of Great Britain, n.12)

THE CHURCH OF ENGLAND

'. . . the foetus has a moral significance insofar as it is potentially a human life and is likely to become a human person in the normal course of events . . .' (*Abortion: An Ethical Discussion*, pp.61-62)

THE BAPTIST UNION OF GREAT BRITAIN AND IRELAND

'After fertilisation, the embryo has the potential to develop into a human being, but until implantation this potential cannot be realised . . .

Until a foetus is viable outside the womb it can only be a *potential* human personality, but it nevertheless deserves respect on precisely that account. . . (There) is clearly an increasing weight of claim to respect as a 'potential personality', as the embryo increases in that potential.' (n.7)

THE METHODIST CHURCH

'There is never any moment from conception onwards when the foetus totally lacks human significance. . . However the degree of this significance manifestly increases.' (*Abortion reconsidered*, n.9)

'Any definition of a person must at least involve reference to an individual being, possessing independence and able to respond to relationships. The foetus progressively develops the potential to exhibit these qualities.' (John Atkinson (edit), *Abortion reconsidered: The Methodist statement and its background,* n.47)

THE CHURCH OF SCOTLAND

'The moral status of the embryo and its moral claim on us do not diminish the further back we go in the stages of its development. From the moment of fertilisation it has the right to be protected and treated as a human being. There is "a serious ambiguity about an argument from the premise that the embryo is 'potentially human', for the potentiality concerned is not that of becoming something else but of becoming what it essentially is." (Prof. T.F. Torrance).' — (1985 General Assembly Report, p.288)

THE CHURCH IN WALES

'The view which seems to be adopted by most people is that of a "sliding scale" of foetal value, that as the foetus develops in the uterus so its intrinsic value increases . . . (There) is at least a degree of difference between the embryo before and the embryo after it is implanted in the womb. . . The step from one to the other appears to be the step from potency for life to actual life. . .To create something with the potential for becoming a human person and develop it solely in order to experiment upon it is to be seen as ethically unacceptable.' (3.9,10 & 12)

There seems to be no disagreement that the 'potency' resides in the embryo itself. To that extent one can understand why the Roman Catholic Archbishops want to insist that it is a 'human being with potential'. However, some of the other churches would feel that this point would be made more accurately by saying that it is a 'human embryo with potential'.

'Potential' demands respect

However the significance of 'potential' is interpreted, there seems to be no disagreement that, since we are dealing with an embryo of the human species, real dignity and reverence is owed to it. This is stated quite clearly even by those churches which do not believe that the embryo is to be given the full respect due to a human being:

THE CHURCH OF ENGLAND

'The foetus, as potentially a human life, has a significance which must not be overlooked, minimised or denied . . . It still remains true that the foetus has a moral significance insofar as it is potentially a human life and is likely to become a human person in the normal course of events. . .' (*Abortion: An Ethical Discussion*, p.61)

'This Synod believes that all human life, including life developing in the womb, is created by God in His own image and is, therefore, to be nurtured, supported and protected.' (Statement to General Synod, 1983)

THE METHODIST CHURCH

'All human life should therefore be reverenced. The foetus is undoubtedly part of the continuum of human existence. . . (The) significance of human life must not be diminished. . . There is never any moment from conception onwards when the foetus totally lacks human significance. . .' (*Abortion reconsidered*, nn.3,7 & 9)

THE BAPTIST UNION OF GREAT BRITAIN AND IRELAND

'Until a foetus is viable outside the womb it can only be a *potential* human personality, but it nevertheless deserves respect on precisely that account . . . (There) is clearly an increasing weight of claim to respect as a "potential personality", as the embryo increases in that potential' (n.7)

THE CHURCH IN WALES

'Even if the embryo has to be treated with respect that does not necessarily mean we have to care for it as if it were an adult human person . . . Our respect for the embryo will increase with its physiological development . . . Although the fertilised embryo deserves respect we are of the opinion that such respect cannot be absolute . . .' (n.3.10,11 & 13)

A human being with potential or a potential human being?

Throughout this chapter I have been careful not to use the phrase 'the dignity of the human person'. That has not been easy since that is the phrase used by virtually everyone today when discussing human rights and human dignity. I have refrained from using that phrase since it seemed to pre-judge the issue of the status of the embryo.

As we have seen, all the churches believe that in some way or other the dignity of the human embryo can only be properly appreciated when seen in the context of reverence for God, our Creator and Redeemer, who is the ultimate foundation of all human dignity. This means that when we are talking about the dignity of the human embryo, it truly is 'human dignity' that we are talking about. Therefore, it also means that just as our reverence for God is involved in our reverence for our fellow human beings, so too is our reverence for God involved in our reverence for the human embryo. Whether our reverence for God is involved in exactly the same way and to the same degree in both cases is the precise issue on which the churches differ. But they do all agree that the human embryo has a God-given dignity which demands our reverence and respect.

The human embryo belongs to the human species. It is alive. Barring accidents and given proper nourishment and the right environment, it will of its own internal dynamism develop progressively into a unique human person whose physical characteristics have been genetically determined from the moment of conception. Even if it were to be proved that its individuality is not definitively established during the earliest days of its existence, it is still an individual being. Therefore, it certainly qualifies for the description 'a living human being'. Its life can accurately be termed 'human life'. All this can be inferred immediately from the empirical evidence.

However, that is not the end of the matter. While this first stage of interpretation leads us to recognise that the human embryo must be treated with reverence, it does not yet answer the question — what kind of reverence? To answer that question demands further reflection and philosophical analysis. It is precisely this analysis which seems to be lacking in the statements of all the churches. The only exception might perhaps be Chapter III of the 1965 Church of England report, *Abortion: An Ethical Discussion*. Without such an analysis the terminology used by the churches hinders rather than helps dialogue.

Is the human embryo 'a human being with potential' or 'a potential human being'? Using the expression 'a human being with potential' is simply making a statement. It does not prove anything. And the same is true of using the other expression 'a potential human being'. These are both short-hand expressions for the conclusion of a long process of analysis and argumentation. Opting for one or other of these expressions, therefore, implies opting for a particular way of analysing and interpreting the phenomenon of being and becoming (or act and potency, as scholastic philosophers would express it). While the churches' differing interpretations of the status of the embryo imply that such an option has been made, the church statements themselves do not attempt to give any explanation of the rationale behind their option. This might be simply an omission on the part of those responsible for the statement. On the other hand, it might be because they have not really analysed the philosophical basis for their option. Unexamined assumptions are a common feature of human discourse. There is no reason to believe that the churches are immune to this aspect of the human condition.

A full philosophical treatment of being and becoming (or act and potency) is outside the scope of this book and I would not be competent to undertake such a task. For the present it is sufficient to note that the major point of division between the churches which differ on this issue seems to be a philosophical question which can be stated as follows: From the point of view of its intrinsic dignity, does a being with potency have the right to exactly the same level of respect and reverence as a being whose potency has been actualised?

If a negative answer is given to that question, another crucial question immediately presents itself. If an equal respect is not the right of a being with potency, just what kind of respect is due to it by right? In other words, how is this respect to be cashed in those instances where it has to be weighed in the balance against other competing claims? This is a question which has not been answered satisfactorily by those churches who, at present, would give a negative answer to the first question.

The 1967 Abortion Act — the churches united against its current operation

All the Christian churches agree that the human embryo demands respect and reverence. That is why the prevalence of abortion in Britain is a matter of grave social concern. The incidence of over two million abortions in this country since the 1967 Abortion Act hardly suggests a prevailing climate of 'reverence' for the human embryo. The Church of Scotland has stated that it is 'appalled' by this fact. The Church of England's General Synod declared in 1983 that it 'views with serious concern the number and consequences of abortions performed in the U.K. in recent years'. The Roman Catholic church has given its full support to organisations working to stem the tide of abortions in Britain.

Abortion is an issue which cannot be left off the agenda in future inter-church dialogue. The Christian churches will be in full agreement that their Christian mission commits them to trying to have a positive influence on public policy and to develop a deeper sense of reverence among people at large. However, they will be greatly impeded in this mission if they are deeply divided among themselves. That is why they must not evade the difficult task of looking together at the status of the embryo. To do this satisfactorily it would appear that the two questions raised above on page 81 must be given high priority on their agenda. And the more basic of these two questions is certainly that concerning the relationship between potency and act. If some kind of agreement could be reached on that question, the kind of 'reverence' due to the human embryo would be easier to discern.

5

What some women are saying about IVF

The essential role of women in Christian theology

I have used the phrase 'some women' quite deliberately in the title of this chapter. That is because its content is based on the views of some women whose writings I have had the opportunity to read. Most of their writing comes from the United States. These women are individuals with their own particular concerns and areas of competence, each approaching the issue of IVF and reproductive medicine with her own personal philosophy of life. What unites them is a common conviction about certain aspects of life. It is this shared conviction which leads them to describe themselves as 'feminists', though they would not want that term to be used oppressively as a rigid definition of a set of beliefs which they must accept as dogma. The label 'feminist' is no more than a helpful short-hand term for describing a way of interpreting experience which many women would share. It is this way of viewing reality that I am referring to throughout this chapter when I use the phrase 'the feminist perspective'.

That the women whose writings are quoted in this chapter differ on specific issues is not surprising; interpreting reality from a feminist perspective in no way implies a uniformity of perception. The feminist perspective is more like a lens through which basic reality is viewed. Individuals will focus that lens differently or will focus it on different aspects of reality. Introducing different depths of focus and changing the angle of vision helps to provide a richer and more comprehensive picture. As a male I am only too pleased to say that my own awareness of what is going on in life has been heightened since I have begun to be introduced to the feminist perspective.

There is little doubt that at present not all women view reality from the feminist perspective. What does seem to be true, however, is that most women, when their eyes are opened to this perspective, feel a sense of liberation. The feminist perspective not only rings true to their own personal experience. It also helps them to accept and own that experience with its various positive and negative features. This in turn enables them to identify the human causes behind some of the negative features and thereby frees them to recognise that human life need not be like this. The human spirit is capable of something better than this.

The unifying elements underlying the rich diversity found in the views of women who would describe themselves as feminist could perhaps be summarised as follows:

(1) The institutions of society have largely been fashioned by men, are predominantly controlled by men, and work primarily for the benefit of men — and the churches would be included among these institutions.

(2) This has resulted in the limitation of the freedom of women and at certain times and in some cultures this limitation of freedom has taken on the form of an oppression which has been more or less barbaric.

(3) One of the major consequences of this situation is that what women have to say has not really been heard or listened to and so the ideas which have been used to shape human culture and interpret human life have been largely the product of men's subjective experience.

(4) Women have something to say which is unique to them as women: this arises partly from the perspective of their experience of oppression and partly from the perspective which is special to them from the very fact that they are women, not men.

I firmly believe that modern feminism, arising as it does out of these four incontrovertible facts, is one of the 'signs of the times'. It is a stirring of the Spirit in our age. If this is true, the Christian church must listen to women, whether they be Christian or not, with very deep respect. The Christian church is in the business of human liberation here on earth, even though it sees the complete fulfilment of that liberation to lie beyond this present life. It sees the finger of God in human affairs wherever true human liberation is taking place. That is why I have not limited myself to listening to the voice of Christian women in this chapter.

The feminist approach is not just restricted to the liberation of women. Setting our world free from the structures of male oppression will bring about not just the liberation of women but the liberation of men also.

> 'Confining this feminine ethic and maternal thinking to merely one sex is damaging for both sexes. In this view, the old saying that "women's liberation means men's liberation" takes a new twist, applying not only to external activity (the liberation of women and men from traditional sex roles and work)

but also to internal styles of thinking, judging and feeling . . . we should all welcome the feminisation of culture.' (Segers 1984, p.249)

The inclusion of this chapter is more symbolic than substantial. Through its inclusion I wish to register my conviction as a man that it is essential that women should play a full part in the debate about IVF. Until this happens in the churches as well, what the churches contribute to the debate will be neither fully Christian nor fully human. It will be only partial — and partiality impedes clear vision. I fully acknowledge that this chapter cannot possibly do justice to what women have to say. Nevertheless, I offer it for what it is worth and I am grateful to all those women who through their writings or personal comments have helped to open my eyes, at least to some extent. I suppose this chapter contains a two-fold request. It is a request to women to continue to make their voice heard. And it is a request to the churches (male-dominated as they all are, though in different ways and to different degrees) to make sure both that the voice of women is heard and that women's ears are fully represented on the official church bodies which have the task of listening to what the Spirit is saying to the churches through women. Until women are properly represented at that level, the official statements of the churches will be defective in their understanding of human life and God's world and consequently the inspiration and guidance they offer will be at best that of the 'partially sighted'.

What is unique about the feminist perspective?

As mentioned earlier, feminists believe that two facets of the experience of women give them a unique perspective on life.

The first is the particular form of oppression that women have experienced as women. In one way or another the oppression of women seems to be universal. It crosses all the boundaries of culture, race, nationality and colour. It is present in religious as well as secular institutions. Its roots seem to go far back into human history and have left their mark deep in the human sub-conscious. It has varied in form and in severity in different countries and in different cultures. In some way or other all women have experienced this oppression, even though not all women may have been aware of it.

Refining the focus of the women's perspective is a task which can only be undertaken by women. The women's perspective is an enriching and challenging gift which women must share with society and with the church. It is an enriching gift since without it reality is viewed only from a male perspective. Such a view is necessarily distorted and out of focus, because reality itself is already disordered by the phenomenon of male domination. 'One challenge that feminists have faced is to convince men and women that beliefs legitimated in male-dominated cultures are just as much the product of men's subjective social experience *as men* as the beliefs produced by women are the product of their social experiences as women.' (Harding 1984, p.209) It is also a challenging gift in that it exposes to view just how crippling to both men and women are many of the social constructs that are based on the distorted male perception of reality.

This first unique element in the feminist perspective will have one overriding question in mind as it investigates IVF and the other forms of reproductive technology. That question is: will this procedure help women to become liberated from the oppression they are currently experiencing or will it merely consolidate that oppression still further?

There is a second element which would seem to be unique about the feminist perspective. Women appear to experience reality differently from men not only because they are oppressed but also because they are women. This fact has often been noted in all sorts of ways down through the ages but it has usually been completely misinterpreted. It has been judged from a male perspective and from that angle women's perception of reality has been found wanting. Consequently, women's experience has been dismissed as fickle, emotional, irrational, subjective etc. Women have been viewed virtually as defective males. Their particular perception of life and human experience has been branded as immature. It is claimed that even such great observers of human experience as Freud and Kohlberg fell into this trap when they came to interpret the experience they had observed. The growing realisation that the women's perspective is an essential and integral part of the rich fabric of human experience is brought out very clearly by Carol Gilligan, *In a Different Voice: Psychological Theory and Women's Development,* (Harvard University Press, Cambridge, Massachusetts and London, 1982). She is implicitly saying that reality will not been seen properly in focus until it is viewed through the twin lenses of women's and men's special perspectives. If this is true, its implications are immense, not least for Christian theology and for the formulation of authoritative Christian statements on matters of belief and practice.

As shall be seen later in the chapter, the feminist perspective, seen from this second angle, focuses principally on our inter-connectedness with each other and therefore on interpersonal responsibility and relationships.

From this perspective, therefore, the question which will predominate in its investigation of IVF and other forms of reproductive technology will be the following: how do these procedures affect our interconnectedness with each other: do they strengthen the web of relationships or do they weaken that web and work in the direction of individualism?

The feminist perspective and abortion

This book is examining different approaches to the ethics of IVF. Part of this examination has involved looking at the abortion issue insofar as it has forced the different churches to clarify their position on the status of the embryo. That is not so with feminists and abortion. Discussion of the status of the embryo has not loomed large in feminist writing on abortion. Nevertheless, the perspective from which they consider abortion is still relevant to an examination of IVF. This is because they see both these practices raising similar questions, which have a bearing on much broader issues affecting society.

Abortion has certainly been a major concern of many feminist writers. Moreover, at least in the United States, most of the 'activists' on both sides of the abortion divide are women. 'Pro-choice' women campaign for the woman's right to choose (i.e. to have her child or to have it aborted); 'pro-life' women campaign for the right to life of the unborn from the moment of conception. However, Kristin Luker's recent sociological survey, *Abortion and the Politics of Motherhood,* (University of California Press, Berkeley, Los Angeles, London, 1984) suggests that the core dispute between the 'pro-choice' and the 'pro-life' activist women is not really about the status of the embryo and its right to life. Rather it is a controversy over different approaches to motherhood and family. 'While on the surface it is the embryo's fate that seems to be at stake, the abortion debate is actually about the meaning of women's lives . . . two opposing visions of motherhood are at war.' (pp.193-194) Theodora Ooms makes the same point when she writes: 'Thus, the abortion controversy, which on first examination appears to be a conflict between two individualistic philosophies, is also, after all, a conflict between two different ideals of family life.' (Ooms 1984, p.101)

However, Luker is at pains to point out that she has only been looking at the 'activists'. Most Americans do not belong to either camp — and presumably that is true also of most women. The more substantial feminist perspective might perhaps be discovered somewhere in the middle ground.

The positions of both the 'pro-choice' and the 'pro-life' activists are related to the 'oppressed' element in the feminist perspective. One is an extreme reaction to the experience of oppression; the other is a counter-reaction from women who may well feel threatened by the call to break loose from the very structures which guarantee them security.

Although some feminist writing would be firmly identified with the pro-choice camp, more and more feminists are beginning to voice criticism of both these extreme positions. This is not a 'middle of the road' feminism, the 'silent majority' suddenly finding its voice. Quite the contrary is true. This is a feminism which refuses to let itself be defined negatively simply in terms of a reaction to male oppression. It owes its origin to the second element in the women's perspective, namely, the belief that women have something special to say *precisely as women*. Hence, it is a feminism which draws its inspiration from the positive experience of women and not just from their negative oppressive experience. Furthermore, it believes that at this stage in history the women's contribution is more important than the men's contribution. This is not because of any intrinsic superiority that their perspective might lay claim to in itself; rather, it is because their perspective has been kept buried for so long that the result has been an increasingly distorted perception of reality.

It is worth examining the critique that this feminist position makes of both the pro-choice and the pro-life activists. It gives a 'feel' for the kind of issues which this same feminist position considers to be important when looking at IVF.

The fundamental criticism is that the 'pro-choice' and the 'pro-life' activists have both been adversely influenced by the increasing individualism of Western society and by the brand of liberal philosophy which undergirds this individualism.

The pro-choice position, for instance, tends to turn the choice of the individual into an absolute. It seems to be based on the vision of the self-sufficient individual who has complete ownership of herself, owing nothing to society and bound by no obligations save those she has chosen to create for herself. Jean Bethke Elshtain relates this to 'a utilitarian ethic and to a perspective that absolutises choice and exalts control at the expense of principles of obligation, human interdependency and caretaking.' (Elshtain 1984, p.49) Moreover, although the pro-choice position claims to be a stance in favour of 'liberation', its critics believe that it ends up by mainly benefitting those with power. This follows from its individualistic basis which fails to pay sufficient attention to the impact of social structures on a person's freedom to choose. Mary B Mahowald writes:

> '. . . the law's insistence on the (practically) exclusive right of the pregnant
> woman to decide the fate of her foetus places a great and ultimately solitary
> burden on many women, some of whom are still children. For that right is not
> one that can be exercised or not; . . . there are surely social factors that greatly
> affect the decision and may severely limit the autonomy of the individual mak-
> ing it. If society were welcoming toward unwed mothers and defective infants
> as well as supportive of the option of abortion in certain cases; if fathers and
> others really shared in child raising; if extra-uterine means of reproduction
> were available; if overpopulation were not a matter of world concern — then we
> would have at least some of the conditions necessary for a genuinely egalitarian
> approach to the abortion issue.' (Mahowald 1984, p.193)

Because abortion on demand promises men 'few restrictions on sexuality and lowers financial responsibility and dependency', feminists like Jean
Bethke Elshtain are not surprised by the statistical evidence which shows
that 'the single group most consistent in favouring an extremely liberal
position on abortion is white upper-middle-class males.' (Elshtain 1984,
p.59) Elshtain also points out that the individualism of the pro-choice
position implies that we are most human when we are in absolute control:
'The irony of the moment may well be that women, caught in the grip of the
rationalist world view, wind up endorsing the image of freedom *from*
nature that, historically, has invited the most insidious forms of domination — of women and of whole ways of life. It is a technocratic prejudice,
not a liberating or democratic ideal, that we are somehow most "human"
when we are in absolute control.' (Elshtain 1984, p.67) This moves in the
direction of technological control over human life. 'Purposeful parenthood' will want the 'perfect child' and so the concept of 'quality control'
moves into human reproduction. This brings with it the implication that
the 'value' of a human life does not come from its intrinsic dignity but is
conferred by others, if the life in question measures up to the requirements
of the consumers choosing it. Whatever good insights feminism draws
from the pro-choice stance, it certainly does not support its implicit option for individualism and the consequences flowing from this option.
Individualism is in stark contrast to the feminist belief in the interconnectedness of all living beings and in the interpersonal responsibilities and
relationships which flow from this.

The pro-life position is also criticised for its individualism. It makes the
rights of the individual its starting-point. As Mary C Segers points out,
'rights language has often proved misleading because the rights that are

stressed are conceived of as being formal, abstract, absolute, and individual — with little attention given to notions of duty and responsibility.' (Segers 1984, p.245) She contrasts this to the findings of Carol Gilligan, after interviewing a number of women contemplating abortion, that 'the feminine construction of the moral domaine relies on a language different from that of men, a language of care and responsibility as opposed to the language of individual rights.' (ibid. p.246)

Many feminists would even regard the 'pro-family' emphasis of the pro-life activists as a disguised form of individualism, a kind of 'family individualism'. They would also criticise it as being far from typical of the experience of most women. Though some women may experience the family as a haven of security, Sandra Harding makes the point that for many the very opposite is true and the family for them is yet another element in the whole social construction of reality which they experience as oppressive. (Harding 1984, pp.214-215)

It is highly significant that the feminist position should makes its principal criticism of both the pro-choice and the pro-life activists the fact that each of them is under the influence of individualism. This supports the contention that they have both allowed themselves to be dominated by the male agenda. Carol Gilligan's research has high-lighted the fact that concentration on the individual pertains to the male way of perceiving reality. (Gilligan 1982, p.62) If Gilligan is right in her analysis of what she calls the 'different voices' of men and women, the criticism of the two extreme activist positions as being too individualistic is implicitly saying that they are speaking more with a 'male voice' than with a 'woman's voice'.

Gilligan believes that the term 'interconnection' provides the key to the way women perceive reality. The lives of all human beings are inter-connected. The fundamental image is that of the 'web'. The web keeps all human beings inter-connected; no one is isolated. Gilligan notes that some men find this image threatening: the web is something that can trap them. The feminist position emphasises relationships and empowerment rather than rules and judgements of condemnation. It focuses more on responsibilities — to others and to oneself — rather than on individual rights to be defended against all comers. It sees the family not just as an intra-personal association but as intergenerational too. Feminist thinking tends to be more contextual and narrative. Issues are not looked at merely in the abstract: they are viewed in their context with all the persons involved, each with his or her own personal story. 'Fair' is a word frequently used when things are seen from the male perspective — 'Is it fair?' 'Care' is the contrasting word used in the feminist perspective — 'How can I show most care in this situation?' The overall flavour of the feminist perspective comes out very clearly in the following passage from Gilligan:

'In this conception, the moral problem arises from conflicting responsibilities rather than from competing rights and requires for its resolution a mode of thinking that is contextual and narrative rather than formal and abstract. This conception of morality as concerned with the activity of care centers moral development around the understanding of responsibility and relationships, just as the conception of morality as fairness ties moral development to the under-standing of rights and rules . . . When asked to describe herself, this woman says that she values "having other people that I am tied to, and also having people that I am responsible to. I have a very strong sense of being responsible to the world, that I can't just live for my enjoyment, but just the fact of being in the world gives me an obligation to do what I can to make the world a better place to live in, no matter how small a scale that may be on." Thus while Kohlberg's sub-ject worries about people interfering with each other's rights, this woman wor-ries about "the possibility of omission, of your not helping others when you could help them."' (ibid. pp.19 & 17)

Seen from this angle, 'mothering' is viewed in a much more positive light by feminists. 'Maternal thinking' is put forward as a feminine trait that women should be anxious to see developing in men: 'Thus, though the practices of mothering are oppressive, at its best, the qualities of mothering or maternal thinking embody the kind of caring we would wish men to express to others. They stand in opposition to the destructive, violent and self-aggrandising characteristics of men.' (Rowland 1985, p.78)

The feminist position I have been describing does not reject the valid insights of the two pro-choice and pro-life activists.

Along with the pro-choice group, it recognises the all-pervasive nature of male oppression. Consequently, it agrees that women must be free to choose. Therefore, it joins ranks with the pro-choice activists to fight against those who would deny freedom of choice to women. In looking at the modern advances in reproductive technology, therefore, it shares the pro-choice concern about the question: do these new procedures work in favour of a woman's right to choose or do they further diminish her freedom of choice?

However, the feminist position does not see the woman's right to choose as absolute. They would argue that a woman should be free to choose as a woman. That means she should be free to consider the situa-tion in all its inter-connectedness, to look at all the relationships involved and the care for herself and others demanded by these relationships, and only then to make her decision. As Mary B Mahowald comments, if this is not recognised and respected, her freedom is being violated:

> 'To treat the pregnant woman as an isolated individual, standing alone in her decision, is insulting in that it strips her of the very context that is integral to her identity. It may be less insulting to define her identity in the limited context of her family. The reality to address, however, is that the pregnant woman stands at the center of multiple social relationships, some of which may be deeper than familial. The fulfillment of her individuality is intimately linked with all such relationships, as well as with her foetus. Her morality is similarly linked with those relationships.' (Mahowald 1984, p.113)

The feminist position, as represented by Mahowald, would claim that this is a 'pro-life' stance in the fullest sense of the term: 'Because life is not lived by individuals in isolation from one another, but as an ongoing, complex system of interpersonal relationships, a really pro-life position does not affirm the life of the foetus alone or the pregnant woman alone; it affirms the life of the community in which they both particpate.' (ibid, p.180)

Feminists stand for 'freedom with responsibility' rather than for absolute and unconditional freedom. Mary C Segers quotes Rosalind Petchesky to great effect on this point:

> 'Recognising a situation of real conflict between the survival of the foetus and the needs of the woman and those dependent on her, the feminist position says merely that women must decide, because it is their bodies that are involved, and because they still have primary responsibility for the care and development of the children born.
>
> But determining who should decide — the political question — does not tell us anything about the moral and social values women ought to bring to this decision, *how* they should decide. Should women get an abortion on the grounds that they prefer a different gender (which amniocentesis can now determine)? Such a decision, in my view, would be blatantly sexist, and nobody's claim to "control of her body" could make it right or compatible with feminist principles. That is, "a woman's right to control her body" is not abstract or absolute, but we have not yet developed a morality . . . that would tell us what the exceptions should be.' (Segers 1984, pp.242-243)

Mahowald is even willing to translate the feminist emphasis on interconnectedness into the more male-orientated language of rights and duties: 'A feminist perspective also reiterates the basic ethical notion that a moral right — for example, the right to control reproduction — involves moral duties. Women who have the legal right to decide also have moral rights and duties to choose responsibly and with consideration for the others affected by reproductive decisions.' (ibid. 245)

Along with the pro-life group, feminists recognise the essential place of the embryo in this whole debate. They accept that the mother (and also the father) is in a relationship of responsibility towards the embryo. In pursuing this point they emphasise that 'inter-connectedness' goes far beyond the realm of human persons. Hence, even if some feminists might not accept the full humanity of the embryo, they would still acknowledge this relationship of responsibility. Naturally, the relative importance given to this particular responsibility will vary according to how the status of the developing embryo is viewed. There is nothing in the feminist position as such which would demand that the full human status of the embryo be either recognised or denied. Consequently, individual feminists will adopt different stances regarding the status of the embryo. Lisa Sowle Cahill, for instance, a Roman Catholic feminist who is both a mother and a professor of moral theology, interprets the status of the embryo as follows:

> 'I am convinced that the foetus is from conception a member of the human species (having an identifiably human genotype, and being of human parentage), and, as such, is an entity to which at least some protection is due, even though its status may not at every phase be equivalent to that of postnatal life. Further, I believe that there exists, even in our pluralist culture, a relatively broad consensus that the foetus does have some value and status in the human community . . . My position on foetal status might be characterised as "developmentalist" insofar as I view its value as incremental throughout gestation . . . Nonetheless, I see the foetus as having a value at conception that is quite significant and that quickly increases; but it never overrides the right of the mother to preserve her own life. Even relatively early in pregnancy (for example, in the first trimester), I think serious considerations must be present to justify abortion. Threat to life is the classic case, although I would not exclude the possibility that other threats might justify abortion, particularly when the interest that the mother has at stake is equal to or greater than her interest in her life.' (Cahill 1984, pp.263-264)

Feminism and the new reproductive technology

How does feminism view the new reproductive technologies? To examine this question in detail, we need to return to the two questions posed earlier in this chapter —

(1) do these new procedures in reproductive technology further the cause of women's liberation from male oppression?

(2) do they enable women to be more truly themselves as women?

It will be helpful to treat these two questions separately.

FIRST QUESTION:

Do the modern advances in reproductive technology further the cause of women's liberation from male domination?

As soon as this question is asked, most feminist writers would insist that it must be properly situated in its real context today. A major factor in that context, they would say, is the way the medical profession intrudes into the lives of women, especially in the very intimate area of their sexual and reproductive faculties. That the medical profession is a bastion of male domination is taken as read by feminist writers, though they would not want to condemn all male doctors by this assertion. Some feminists have written very revealingly about the way many women feel that their male doctors are simply incapable of taking them seriously when, for instance, they complain about the side-effects of medical treatment or contraceptive measures. One feminist writer, Scarlet Pollock, expresses it thus: 'Medical dominance, accentuated by male dominant perceptions of women, resulted in frequent conflicts between women and their doctors. Convincing her doctor that she is a rational and responsible human being, and not "another neurotic female", is not always an easy task for a woman.' (Pollock 1984, p.143) Renate Duelli Klein puts it even more strongly: 'Women's desires and needs, our experiences of our own bodies, are discredited and declared neurotic and hysterical or simply part of the "disease" of being female.' (Klein 1985, p.67)

Consequently, feminists have a suspicion of any further medical intrusion into the woman's reproductive role. Some feminists even voice the fear that modern reproductive technology is enabling men to deprive women of their natural reproductive role. Julie Murphy argues that this is suggested by the very language which is used among reproductive technicians: 'The scientific term, "egg recovery", refers to the removal of eggs from women's bodies. Yet for women, "egg recovery" is a misnomer. "Recovery" implies prior attachment or ownership. One recovers something one once lost control of or misplaced. When eggs are taken out of women's bodies, however, women do not recover anything. Women lose something, namely, eggs. It is patriarchy that "recovers" or possesses the eggs.' (Murphy 1984, p.70)

Janice Raymond in her Preface to *Man-Made Women: How new reproductive technologies affect women,* (Hutchinson, London, 1985) sums up what would seem to be the concerns and fears of many women who have tried to think through the deeper implications of developing reproductive technologies as seen in their true context within the contemporary medical scene:

'Perhaps the most confusing message about the new reproductive technologies is that they are a gift to women, because they appear to give so-called infertile women the ability to reproduce. However, when women look this "gift-horse" in the mouth, they will see that it comes accompanied by the persistent *medicalisation* of women's lives. This means that more and more areas of female living have been colonised by medical intervention, and staked out as medical territory. The medicalisation of female existence, begun with the nineteenth-century establishment of the specialities of gynaecology and obstetrics, becomes outrageously solidified in the new technologies of reproduction. Obscured by all the recent accounts of the "miracles" of reproductive technologies is the immense amount of biomedical probing, manipulation, and experimentation to which women who seek out such "wonders" of technological fertility and birthing are subject.' (Corea, p.12)

This developing awareness among women is also causing some feminists to have misgivings even about certain aspects of contraception. Feminists have often seen this as an area where freedom of choice seemed to be working more unambiguously in favour of women's liberation. Now, however, serious doubts are being expressed about the effect of the contraceptive pill. (cf. Rowland 1985, pp.80-81)

There is another crucial issue which is high-lighted by feminist writers considering the impact of reproductive technologies on women's liberation. This is the theme of 'social control'. Barbara Katz Rothman is a feminist writer who has consistently looked at this theme in her writings:

'While technology opens up some choices, it closes down others. The new choice is often greeted with such fanfare that the silent closing of the door on the old choice goes unheeded . . . While on the one hand we worry, with very good reason, about losing the option of legal abortions, on the other hand we are losing the option not to abort . . . This woman who kept her fourth pregnancy made a choice, but it is a choice which may be rapidly slipping away from us. She is suffering not just the inevitable consequences of four children, but the consequences of her poverty. If she was rich, if her husband made a fortune, she would still be tired, I'm sure, but she would have many more choices in how she lives her life as the mother of four young children.

The choice of contraception simultaneously closed down some of the choices for large families. North American society is geared to small families, if indeed to any children at all . . .

Choices open and choices close. For those whose choices meet the social expectations, for those who want what the society wants them to want, the experience of choice is very real.

Perhaps what we should realise is that human beings living in society have precious little choice ever. There may really be no such thing as individual choice in a social structure, not in any absolute way. The social structure creates needs — the needs for women to be mothers, the needs for small families, the needs for 'perfect' children — and creates the technology which enables people to make the needed choices. The question is not whether choices are constructed, but how they are constructed. Society, in its ultimate meaning, may be nothing more and nothing less than the structuring of choices.' (Rothman 1984, pp.24, 27-28, 32)

In the light of her analysis, Rothman is led to the conclusion: 'The question then for feminism is not only to address the individual level of "a woman's right to choose" but also to examine the social level, where her choices are structured.' (ibid, p.32)

Some feminists would go even further than Rothman and say that what will soon be at stake will be a woman's right to have a child of her own: 'Among the things the next "wave" of the women's movement might have to fight for, could be a woman's right to bear our own natural children: we could have lost control over the last part of the reproductive process: to decide if, when, and how to conceive, carry and give birth to children.' (Klein 1985, p.71) This ties in with the incredible fact that in the United States a child (if disabled, for instance) could sue its mother for 'wrongful birth' because she did not have it aborted!

This concern about 'social control' is an absolutely basic theme in the whole feminist movement. The deep hostility towards the take-over of reproductive functioning by the medical profession is but one instance of a much deeper social critique which has been latent in most feminist positions but which is being increasingly articulated. Its radical social and political implications are being explored very thoroughly by many contemporary feminist writers.

It is at this level that the feminist position is seen most clearly as a movement not just for women's liberation but for human liberation. From this angle the feminist analysis reveals that the same causes are at work in women's oppression as are operative in all the other forms of human oppression. Sandra Harding brings this out well in her analysis of the abortion issue:

> 'What I perceive as the distinctively women's issues in the abortion dispute could transform the feminist political agenda, thereby revealing the illegitimacy of the entire social order . . .the presence of the abortion issue on the public agenda can reveal to women what has often been hidden from our understanding: Issues of who should control sexuality and reproduction and of how it should be controlled are inextricably linked with the broadest economic, political, and social issues about what kinds of persons we want to be and what we want human social life to look like.
>
> . . . The importance of the feminist agenda is that it focuses on how both sexes are fully human, it explores how the sexual order is a fundamental component of the social order, and it dismantles the edifices build on the assumption that *human* goals, desires, and ways of structuring social relations are identical with the masculine forms of these goals, desires, and relations.' (Harding 1984, pp.223-224)

Sandra Harding's comments lead us naturally to look at the second question which has to be faced.

SECOND QUESTION:

Do the modern advances in reproductive technology enable women to be more truly themselves as women?

The first way into this question is an indirect one. It is through trying to interpret the phenomenon of 'social control' that has been high-lighted by so many women.

As feminist writers have pointed out, the dominant social philosophy that seems to be influencing most Western societies is a form of liberal individualism. The hollowness of the individual freedom that this claims to bring about in society is shown up by women like Harding and Rothman who expose the powerful effects of social control on people's lives. In fact, social control is a form of *power*. It is a subtle form of power working to further the interests of the group in whose favour society is primarily organised. Whether consciously or unconsciously, the fundamental institutions of society (political, legal, education, medical and even ecclesiastical) all serve this purpose. To keep peace in society other interests are catered for as far as possible. However, in the case of a conflict of interest, the power structures tend to work in favour of those whose interests are being principally served by society. When such a conflict arises, the exercise of power becomes more evident and it is experienced more directly as oppression. It tends to work on two levels. The cost of society's not being able to serve all interests is borne mainly by those whose interests take second place. In this situation, the very structures of society are experienced by these second-class citizens as working against their favour. This becomes concrete in terms of cut-backs in health care and welfare provision, educational cuts, unemployment etc. And when the violence experienced through these oppressive measures provokes protest (whether violent or non-violent) among those who are paying the cost of society's ills, power is then exercised in the form of suppression of dissent. This latter exercise of power often operates under the guise of law and order enforcement to safeguard the common good.

The above paragraph might seem to be a rather naive, left-wing, revolutionary analysis which is totally irrelevant to the issues we are considering. I do not think that is true. The women's movement is not just one instance of the voice of the power-less, though it is that, of course. What makes it essentially different is the fact that *from the feminist perspective* one of the principal ills of societies like ours is precisely their reliance on *power* as the principal instrument for shaping society and solving human conflict. The feminist perspective sees power as pertaining to the male way of approaching reality and as such it is a profound distortion of human reality. Helen Holmes and Betty Hoskins bring this out in their examination of sex choice technologies:

> 'the real heart of the problem is that sex choice technologies would nurture patriarchy. All current forms of government are patriarchal: they foster competitiveness and have hierarchies of power and privilege; "masculine" traits, such as aggressiveness, are rewarded. "Feminine" qualities, such as compassion and co-operation, are disparaged. The earth, seen as feminine, is exploited. (The term "patriarchal" does not necessarily mean "male"; there are patriarchal women, and non-patriarchal men.) We believe that this patriarchal attitude towards the living and non-living earth, the weak, the poor, the "others", is at the root of all the problems that are threatening the very existence of human life on this planet: poverty, pollution, nuclear war, and yes, over-population.' (Holmes & Hoskins 1985, p.23)

As long as power is the dominant motif, feminists mistrust the various forms of reproductive technology. They are viewed as yet one more weapon in the armoury of oppressive instruments which can be wielded against the true interests of women. In a different kind of society altogether, they might be welcomed, insofar as they were seen to be increasing the opportunites and possibilities of relationship and caring among all the members, male and female, of society.

Apart from this general point, are there any specific points made precisely from the women's perspective vis-à-vis the new reproductive technologies?

One aspect of reproductive technology to which the feminist perspective has paid special attention is the issue of sex-selection. The strongest condemnation of sex-selection comes from Tabitha Powledge who describes it as 'the original sexist sin' and who says it 'is one of the most stupendously sexist acts in which it is possible to engage.' (Holmes & Hoskins 1985, p.23)

Why is there such strong feeling among feminists on this issue? Research has shown that, given the choice, the vast majority of people would choose to have a son as their first-born child. One study conducted in 1983 showed that from a group of college students '81% of the women and 94% of the men preferred firstborn sons'. (Steinbacher & Holmes 1985, p.56) Often when sex-selection is discussed, the major concern expressed is whether it might affect the natural numerical balance of the sexes. Feminist writers, while not discounting the fears voiced regarding numbers, turn their attention more to its effect on the status of women. They stress the fact that widespread sex-selection will mean that daughters, when chosen, will be 'planned-to-be-second'. They also note that the case for sex-selection is normally argued on the grounds that it extends freedom of choice and this will benefit the child since it will be a 'wanted' child in a much fuller sense. Some feminists believe that the reality is likely to be quite different. The advantage of knowing that they were 'wanted' in this way could be completely negated for girls by the knowledge that they were wanted as 'second' to their brothers. As Steinbacher remarks: 'The *de facto* second class status of women in the world would be confirmed *in fact, by choice.*' (quoted in Holmes & Hoskins 1985, p.22) She makes this point even more forcefully in her joint article with Helen B Holmes:

> 'Individually, when females realise that they are chosen to be second, the psychological ramifications will be incalculable. The notion of inferiority which society still dictates for women as a class, despite the women's movement, undoubtedly would be further internalised and externalised. The sharply reduced numbers of females when they come to be chosen for reproductive purposes or to be little sisters, may well be regarded (by themselves and by others) as 'chosen' for powerlessness.' (Steinbacher & Holmes 1985, p.60)

This concern of the feminist perspective is virtually ignored in the church statements I have examined. The Roman Catholic Bishops' Joint Committee on Bio-Ethical Issues express opposition to sex-selection but only on the grounds that it will probably entail the destruction of embryos. (cf. Evidence nn.13 & 27 and Response n.43) Some of the working party which produced the Church of England report, *Personal Origins,* are opposed to sex-selection because 'the sex of our children is something to be received by us, not to be determined by us'. The rest of the working party see 'no basic moral problems' with it 'provided it is possible to organise and manage such choices in an acceptable manner.' (n.131) The only church report I have seen which pays particular attention to the social consequences of sex-selection is the evidence submitted to the Warnock Committee by the Social Welfare Commission of the Roman Catholic Bishops' Conference. However, its conclusion shows that even it does not share the fears of the feminist perspective:

> 'We do not foresee obvious, unwelcome social consequences. Imbalance of sexes in the general population seems self-adjusting over a period of time. In Western society, at least, it seems unlikely that there would develop such a preference on the part of parents for one particular sex that the State would need to consider remedial measures.' (n.31)

The Warnock Report itself is more alert to the dangers high-lighted by some feminist writers but even that Report was unable to make any positive recommendations on the issue. (9.11)

Little imagination is needed to appreciate what sex selection might mean in those countries where a male child assumes such importance that women are obliged to abort their female offspring, if they are not to be rejected by their husbands. (Roggencamp 1984, pp.266-277 and Kishwar 1985, pp.30-37) and where the practice of 'fatal forms of neglect of female children is widely prevalent' and is used as a substitute for the now outlawed practice of 'female infanticide'. (Kishwar 1985, p.31)

The point is also made that, the pressures of social control working in the way they do, women may be in danger of losing the right not to choose the sex of their child. (Rowland 1985, p.85)

The feminist perspective also points out that the increasing invasion of the 'quality control' mentality into the field of human reproduction is likely to have a serious negative impact on the child's feeling 'accepted' by its parents. This could have a devastating effect on a child's psychological and emotional development. Jean Bethke Elshtain writes:

'The technocratic world view buttresses the human arrogance that it may soon be possible for couples to aim for the perfect child. One could, in this image, abort all less-than-perfect models (as revealed through a panoply of tests). Should the one perfect child turn out, as all children must, to be less than perfect, it bodes ill for parent-child relations. More important, what is at stake here is our human capacity for risk taking, spontaneity, and welcoming.' (Elshtain 1984, p.69)

Barbara Katz Rothman makes the same point even more simply: 'It seems that, in gaining the choice to control the quality of our children, we may be losing the choice not to control the quality, the choice of simply accepting them as they are.' (Rothman 1984, p.30; cf. also Rothman 1985, pp.188-193)

The feminist perspective also enables the issue of commercial surrogate motherhood to be seen in a new light. In ethical discussions on this matter surrogacy is normally rejected for two reasons, each of them involving an implicit condemnation of the surrogate mother herself: she is demeaning herself as a woman and it is wrong for her to make money in this way. The women's perspective accepts the prostitution model as applied to commercial surrogacy but, being more ready to see a prostitute as a 'victim' rather than as a moral reprobate, feminist writers see the 'reproductive prostitute' in this light also. In fact, the plight of some of the surrogate mothers involved provides an extreme example of the exploitation of women in the market place of the reproductive industry:

'It is a myth that women are easily making large sums of money as surrogates. The director of this program acknowledges that the woman who goes through a lengthy insemination process may end up being paid less than $1.00/hour for her participation. To earn this sum, she is completely 'on call' for the company. She may be required to undergo invasive diagnostic procedures, forfeit her job, and perhaps undergo major surgery with its attendant morbidity and mortality risks. Of course, should there be a miscarriage or failure to conceive, the surrogate receives no compensation at all.' (Ince 1984, pp.111 & 115)

Even more horrifying is the very real possibility that the surrogacy industry will begin to operate at an international level and thereby consolidate still further the oppression of women in the Third World. Gena Corea writes: 'When it becomes possible to transfer human embryos routinely from one woman to another (and it has already been done experimentally), then the way opens up to use Third World women to gestate babies for wealthier westerners'. She goes on to report:

'The president of a US foundation which helps arrange surrogate pregnancies told me: "If we could cross international lines, then $1000 is a significant sum of money, whereas here (in the US), it's just a week or a month's wages." Asked what countries he had in mind, he replied: "Central America would be fine." It is "inevitable" that the United States go to other parts of the world and "rely on their support" in providing surrogate mothers, he thinks. Comparing the United States to the city and Central America to the country, he pointed out that "the cities are always supported by the country".' (Corea 1985, pp.43-44)

This links with a further point made by feminist writers, namely, that women, especially in poorer countries, are virtually being used for experimental purposes to try out the effectiveness of new forms of reproductive medicine, particularly in the field of contraception. (Rowland 1985, p.75; cf. also Klein 1985, p.68)

Finally, the point is made by some feminist writers that the advent of modern technology in the field of human procreation can serve to consolidate the sexually oppressive view that a woman needs to be a mother if she is to be truly a woman in the full sense of the word. This functional view of women has strongly influenced the Christian church from its earliest days. Even St Augustine, generally acknowledged to be the greatest theologian in the first millenium of the Christian church, was affected by this view:

'If woman has not been made for helping man by bearing children, what other kind of help can she give? Not manual labour, since another man is much better help than a woman; not for the sake of company if a man is feeling lonely, because another man is much better company and you can have a much more worthwhile conversation with a man than with a woman; not even for the sake of having people in society who are by nature submissive to men and who will obey orders — men have shown they do that just as well as women, if order in society demands it! So honestly, I do not know what is the point of God's making woman if it is not for the sake of bearing children.' (St Augustine, *De Gen.*, ad litt, IX n.5 *CSEL*, XXXVIII — my own translation)

Rebecca Albury voices the fear of feminists that 'the unquestioned availability of technological conception could provide increased pressure on women to conform to the definition of femininity that requires motherhood.' (Albury 1984, p.63)

Conclusion

In previous chapters we have examined the differing approaches of the

Christian churches regarding the new procedures in reproductive medicine and technology. It is interesting to note the contrast between these church statements and the women's perspective.

By and large, the church bodies have concentrated on such issues as — the status of the foetus, the needs of the infertile couple, the welfare of the child, the nature of the sexual act and how far God's design can be found written into the order of nature. The question as posed by the churches has been: is IVF morally acceptable? Moreover, in linking this question to the status of the embryo they have felt forced to take up positions on a question of *rights*. The Roman Catholic church has opted for the rights of the unborn. The other churches, to varying degrees, give more weight to the rights of the mother and her family. But it has been a 'rights' issue for both groups.

The women's perspective has a somewhat different 'feel' about it. The focus is less on abstract questions that need to be resolved. Rather one gains the impression that women are sensing that something is *happening* here which could be unhealthy for humanity. They are not trying to provide answers for abstract questions so that these answers can then regulate human conduct. Instead they are looking at the wider context and are trying to listen to human experience in order to discern what is going on and how it might be affecting the whole web of human life and relationships. Whereas the pro-choice activists are campaigning on a 'rights' issue (the woman's right to choose), the mainstream feminist writers seem to be viewing the whole matter from a different perspective to that of individual rights. One detects a feeling of 'concern' about how this new technology is affecting *people,* particularly women, in our society.

It would be unfair to exaggerate this point. There is plenty of 'care and concern' evident in many of the church statements and likewise the feminist writers are far from ignoring the important philosophical issues. However, in the main the church reports seem closer to what Carol Gilligan would describe as 'the male voice'. The church document which seems to incorporate more of 'the female voice' is the report, *Choices in Childlessness,* produced by a joint Working Party of the Free Church Federal Council and the British Council of Churches. It is interesting to note that there was an equal number of men and women on that Working Party. That was not the case with the *Personal Origins* Working Party which was made up of four men and one woman, nor with the Roman Catholic Bishops' Joint Committee on Bio-Ethical Issues which comprised thirteen men and four women.

The well-being of women is not top priority on the feminist agenda. Their top priority is 'caring' for the whole human family:

> 'The power which microbiology and biomedicine has given to us to regulate and interfere with the reproduction of the species requires, if we wish to retain our humanity, that we rethink what it is we are about, what we value in each other, children, women and men, and how in the new circumstances we can achieve those values . . . Most discussions one hears today, for example about *in vivo* or *in vitro* fertilisation or gene therapy, are conducted in terms of reducing the suffering of individuals. This is not surprising because clinical medicine has always been individualistic, treating the pain, the suffering, the pathology which is presented by individuals. In the area of the new reproductive technology this is not enough. There are immense social consequences going far beyond the individual case . . . We have to think . . . at the social level and see children as a collective joy and responsibility rather than as private property, our own or anyone else's.' (Stacey 1985, p.194)

If the agenda of the churches is to be properly influenced by the feminist perspective, much more is needed than a slot on the agenda for 'women's issues'. It needs to be recognised that at present all the issues being discussed are being seen from a 'partial' point of view. All these issues need to be properly focused so that they can be seen through the twin lenses of the male and female perspective. The very act of focusing involves fusing together what is unique to each perspective.

6

Dialogue and self-criticism
A Roman Catholic first step

Pointing out weaknesses in another person's position is a valid exercise in the context of dialogue. However, unless it is accompanied by a willingness to be self-critical as well, it can easily turn dialogue into confrontation and polemics. The same is true at a community level and between communities. Consequently, it seems important for inter-church dialogue on ethical issues that the different churches should be willing to be self-critical of their own positions, when necessary. This is not easy when one is involved in dialogue as a representative of one's church, since to raise questions about the position of one's own church can sometimes be interpreted almost as a betrayal or a lack of loyalty to one's church. Yet to ignore legitimate questions that need to be asked can show a lack of confidence in the good faith of one's own church and can even betray one's own personal commitment to truth. Of its very nature dialogue is about a common search for truth.

Vatican II was a tremendously courageous and far-reaching exercise of this kind of self-criticism within the Roman Catholic church. Pope Paul VI, in his opening discourse for the Council's second session, said that the Church's 'primary duty' in Vatican II was 'to reform, correct and set herself aright in conformity with her divine model'. (quoted in Congar 1964, p.51)

Within the Roman Catholic church, on ethical issues moral theologians have an important role to play in this exercise of constructive self-criticism. Speaking of their role, Karl Rahner writes:

'. . . it is also the task of academic moral theology, not only to expose as such what is unproved in the course of the argument, but also to work to break down the preconceptions behind it, if these are themselves historically conditioned and no longer correspond to the concrete "reality" they are meant to support and which they reproduce without further consideration. This is a difficult task for which the Church's magisterium with its conservative attitude (understandable but perhaps also unjustified) generally shows little gratitude.

. . . the moral theologian cannot be merely the interpreter and defender of the traditional teaching of the magisterium, but also its critic who helps the magisterium to understand better and more effectively to defend before humanity the teaching of Christian revelation and of man's self-understanding in the history of his morality.' (*Theological Investigations*, vol 18, pp.80-81)

I have written this chapter as a small contribution to the dialogue from the Roman Catholic side. I have written it on the assumption that the Roman Catholic position would not want to claim that it has said the final word on the issue. Consequently, I believe that the truth will best be served if that position can be further refined or formulated more adequately, if that is seen to be necessary. I am also working on a similar assumption that the other churches would also be open to the possibility that their positions might also be in need of refinement or re-formulation. I could have written a further chapter containing a critical analysis of the positions of the other churches. I have deliberately refrained from doing that in the hope that this present chapter will be seen as an invitation to the other churches to undertake that task themselves. Criticisms from the outside are heard more sympathetically after we have been prepared to undertake our own internal task of self-criticism.

FIRST QUESTION

How far is the Roman Catholic position on contraception a determining factor in its assessing the morality of IVF?

As mentioned in Chapter 1, there is some division of opinion on this point in the Roman Catholic church in Britain. The 'majority' position of the Catholic Bishops' Joint Committee on Bio-Ethical Issues judges IVF to be 'morally flawed' because it severs procreation from intercourse. The Bishops' Conference of England and Wales, on the other hand, 'see no reason to consider "the simple case" of IVF, as morally unacceptable', though they later qualify this statement and hint that 'the Church's teaching concerning marital intercourse as the proper context for the transmission of human life' might pose 'serious questions' for IVF. Presumably neither of these bodies rejects the Roman Catholic teaching on contraception.

What are we to make of this?

It might be argued that IVF is not a mirror-image of contraception. To maintain that the sexual act is intrinsically immoral when its openness to life is deliberately excluded is to say nothing about procreation itself and how it should be brought about.

At a surface level that is true. However, whether it is true at a much deeper level depends on the fundamental argument put forward for rejecting contraception. The rejection of contraception is a conclusion, not a premise. The basic premise from which the Roman Catholic church draws this conclusion seems to have two elements within it, both of which are viewed as 'God-given': (1) the inseparability of the unitive and procreative 'goods' of marriage; and (2) the deeply symbolic embodiment of these inseparable 'goods' within marriage found in the couple's use of their sexual faculties.

To accept this basic premise would seem to imply the rejection of both contraception and IVF since it is saying not simply that these two 'goods' must never be separated from each other but also that the only locus where God has intended them to be kept together is in the couple's use of their sexual faculties. In the case of contraception, the unitive is separated from the procreative *within* the sexual act; in the case of IVF, the procreative is separated from the unitive *outside* the sexual act. However, both offend against the same basic principle which states that the unitive and the procreative are inseparable and that their inseparability is enshrined within the use of our sexual faculty. It is not simply a matter of respecting this inseparability whenever the sexual act is performed, as though what happened outside the sexual act was a different matter altogether, thus leaving procreation outside the sexual act an open question. The Roman Catholic teaching maintains that we are only respecting the God-given order of creation when we keep the unitive and the procreative inseparable from each other and within their God-given exclusive locus which is the use of our sexual faculties within marriage.

Pius XII was quite clear about this when he dealt with the issue of artificial insemination. In an address to Catholic Doctors (29 September 1949) he said:

'Although new methods cannot be excluded *a priori* merely because they are new, nevertheless, as regards artificial insemination, it is not enough to be extremely reserved, it must be absolutely excluded. Saying this does not necessarily proscribe the use of certain artificial means destined solely to facilitate the natural act, or to assure the accomplishment of the end of the natural act normally performed.

Only the procreation of a new life according to the will and design of the Creator — and never let this be forgotten — brings with it, in a wonderful degree of perfection, the fulfilment of the proposed ends. It is, at the same time, in conformity with bodily and spiritual nature and the dignity of husband and wife, as well as the normal and healthy development of the child.'

In repeating the same teaching in his address to Catholic midwives (29 October 1951), he makes it clear that he rejects artificial insemination because he believes in the personal/relational character of the marital act:

> 'To consider unworthily the cohabitation of husband and wife and the marital act as a simple organic function for the transmission of seed, would be the same as to convert the domestic hearth, which is the family sanctuary, into a mere biological laboratory. For this reason, in Our Address . . . to the International Congress of Catholic Doctors, We formally rejected artificial insemination in marriage . . . (The marital act) is much more than union of two life-germs, which can be brought about even artificially, that is, without the co-operation of the husband and wife. The marital act, in the order of, and by nature's design, consists of a personal cooperation. . .'

The point Pius XII is stressing is that only when procreation comes about as the result of such a personal/relational act can it be said to be 'carried out according to the will and plan of the Creator'. Pius XII was even more explicit in his address to the 2nd World Congress on Fertility and Sterility (19 May 1956). There he condemns artificial contraception and immediately goes on to condemn artificial insemination for the same basic reason:

> 'And the Church has likewise rejected the opposite attitude that would pretend to separate, in generation, the biological activity from the personal relation of the marriage couple. The child is the fruit of the conjugal union when that union finds full expression by bringing into play the organic functions, the associated sensible emotions and the spiritual and disinterested love that animates it. It is within the unity of this human activity that the biological pre-requisites of generation should take place.'

In the same address Pius XII goes on to reject IVF experiments: 'On the subject of experiments in artificial human fecundation "in vitro", let it suffice for us to observe that they must be rejected as immoral and absolutely illicit.' Moreover, the reason he gives for this condemnation is once again the violation of the inseparability of the procreative and unitive 'goods' which should be preserved intact in their God-given locus of the marital act:

> 'Artificial fertilisation goes beyond the limits of the right which the spouses have acquired through the marriage contract, namely, the right to fully exercise their natural sexual capacity within the natural performance of the marriage act. Their marriage contract does not confer on them the right to artificial fertilisation, for such a right is in no way included in the right to the natural marriage

act nor can it be deduced from it. Still less can it be derived from the right of the child as the primary end of marriage. The marriage contract does not give this right, because its object is not the "child" but the "natural acts" which are capable of generating a new life and which are destined for this.'

Richard McCormick, in his article *Therapy or Tampering? The Ethics of Reproductive Technology* (*America*, 7/12/85) notes that this line of argument is still current in Roman Catholic discussions of IVF and he remarks on its intrinsic link to the basic premise from which the Roman Catholic condemnation of contraception is drawn:

'This is still the position taken by some within the Catholic community. Thus the Catholic bishops of Victoria, Australia, in submitting their opinion (1983) to the Waller Committee, stated: "In pursuit of the admirable end of helping an infertile couple to conceive and have their baby, IVF intervenes in their supreme expression of mutual love. It separates 'baby-making' from 'love-making'." Similarly, Mgr Carlo Caffarra, head of the Pontifical Institute for the Family, appeals to the inseparability of the unitive and the procreative to reject IVF. "The moral problem is that procreation can no longer be said to be — and in fact is not — dependent upon the sexual act between two married people." Were theologians like Caffarra to approve of IVF, they would have to allow some separation of the unitive and the procreative — and thus forfeit the basis for Pope Paul VI's and Pope John Paul II's rejection of contraception.' (pp.398-399)

It is worth noting that the prominent Australian Jesuit moral theologian, William Daniel, does not share the view of the Catholic bishops of Victoria. He argues (unconvincingly, to my mind) that IVF can be justified according to the principles enunciated in *Humanae Vitae*:

'If Paul VI could argue that the reason *contraception* is wrong is because it is not true to the relationship that the act is seeking to express, could it not be argued that IVF is an attempt to express that relationship, and certainly not a contradiction of it? I am not trying to argue from the goodness of the end that is being sought. I am suggesting that IVF is an act *true to the marriage relationship*, contradicting neither of the elements that Paul VI proposed as essential. The "union of bodies" that we associate with procreation becomes here metaphorical, but the "mutual self-giving" to which Pius XII has referred is being achieved through the medium of the gametes which the husband and wife have contributed from their own bodies for the fertilisation of the ovum.' (Daniel, 1984, p.62)

In a footnote he adds a comment which seems rather similar to the position of the Hierarchy of England and Wales: 'In this context I would suggest that the teaching of *Humanae Vitae* should be understood *affirmative sed non exclusive* about the qualities of the sexual act. In other words, it teaches that if the sexual act is performed it should have these qualities. This does not logically imply that if one is to have procreation it must be by the performance of the unitive act.' (*op.cit.* p.70, n.35)

For McCormick himself there is no doubt as to what is the basic issue in this whole discussion:

> 'The issue at stake should be clear: the meaning of the inseparability of the unitive and the procreative. Specifically, must these be held together in *every act* (thus no contraception or IVF), or is it sufficient that the *spheres* be held together, so that there is no procreation apart from marriage, and no full sexual intimacy apart from a context of responsibility of procreation? As long as there is debate on these understandings, IVF will be as controversial as Pope Paul VI's encyclical *Humanae Vitae.*' (p.399)

I fully agree with McCormick on this point. I fail to see how the basic grounding of the Roman Catholic position on contraception does not also necessarily involve the rejection of IVF. Of course, that does not imply that IVF automatically becomes justified once the acceptability of responsible contraception in marriage is granted. As we have seen from the positions of the different churches, there are other substantial objections raised to IVF. As the position of Oliver O'Donovan demonstrates (cf. supra, p.24) accepting responsible contraception within marriage would not even necessarily imply an 'in principle' acceptance of IVF.

Maybe the fact that there is division within the British Roman Catholic church on this point indicates that by way of preparation for any inter-church dialogue on IVF it would need to be more fully discussed within the Roman Catholic community. However, if McCormick's view is correct, there will be no possibility of any worthwhile inter-church dialogue on IVF if the basic premise underlying the Roman Catholic position on contraception is not included for discussion on the agenda. To facilitate that, my second point of Roman Catholic self-criticism looks at that precise issue.

SECOND QUESTION

Contraception re-visited

The Roman Catholic position on artificial contraception is bound up with our understanding of what is meant by the natural law. Consequently, this section will examine how Roman Catholic moral theologians today understand natural law and how far this understanding ties in with the teaching of Vatican II and *Humanae Vitae*.

THE NATURAL LAW AND WHAT IS NATURAL

Whether an action is in accord with our God-given nature or not has nothing directly to do with whether that action is artificial or not. *Choices in Childlessness* makes this point very well:

> '. . . the popular ethical distinction between the "natural" and the "unnatural" is a distinction between what is in keeping with human nature and what is not. It is not a distinction between the natural and the artificial. Since, then, human beings are by nature intelligent and creative, and the adaptation of the environment to their needs is an expression of their intelligence, human artifice, such as that developed in medical technology, is in principle ethically natural.' (p.42)

It is precisely this ethical meaning of 'natural' that most Roman Catholic moral theologians would have in mind today when they speak of the 'natural law'. Moreover, in this they would see themselves as being substantially faithful to the basic Thomistic understanding of natural law. How they would understand natural law is well explained by Joseph Fuchs, one of the most respected Roman Catholic moral theologians writing today:

> 'The fact that man — as the image of God (Gen 1) — is a *person* means not merely that he can accept, preserve, contemplate mankind, the world of men and himself as a given reality, but rather that he should grasp it, have control over it, shape it, develop it, increasingly and in a more active fashion stamp it with his own nature — in other words increasingly "humanise" it. Man and his world are not simply actuality, but also potentiality; the given reality and possible development are a single actuality and are in the charge of man as created person-in-world. As person-in-world, man has to make an ever fresh attempt to discover in what way man's conduct, the formation of human society and the control and "utilisation" of the reality of the world in the service of mankind can be truly human, can measure up to the dignity of man as a person in this reality. In other words; what kind of progress can be called "human" progress in the true sense of the word? *In so far as he discovers this correctly, he arrives at a knowledge of the natural law.*
>
> Natural law . . . cannot be read from facts of nature as though God had woven it into them; for all that can be read from the facts of nature are physical data and laws, not moral regulations and commands. The natural moral law is

rather to be understood in a dynamic sense; as the ever new and still to be solved problem of being a person of this world . . .

The norm of correct moral behaviour cannot simply be found in the fact of its conformity with physical nature as such, but rather in its conformity with the human person taken in his totality — not, therefore, without regard for the peculiarity of purely physical nature . . . Thus it is not the physical law that has to be considered as a moral law and invoked to regulate the free actions of mankind, but the "recta ratio" which understands the person in the *totality* of his reality. . .

. . . Is it permitted to touch upon the reality of man? . . . It would certainly be false to say — because God has created man as he finds himself to be in actuality, therefore this is the best manner of existence for men. For God has created man *complete with the possibility of his development,* and indeed of his self-development. This is therefore man's duty even though we may have difficulties in recognising which transformation of man represents a true human value. But fundamentally we ought not to be afraid of touching upon the reality of man. On the contrary, this is our duty precisely because man, with these possibilities, is dependent upon God his Creator.' (Fuchs 1970, pp.182-183, 184, 143 & 117)

VATICAN II AND NATURAL LAW

This understanding of the natural law, which would be accepted by most Roman Catholic moral theologians, ties in with a key passage from Vatican II, dealing with the birth control issue:

'When there is question of harmonising conjugal love with the responsible transmission of life, the moral aspect of any procedure does not depend solely on sincere intentions or on an evaluation of motives. It must be determined by objective standards. These, based on the nature of the human person and his acts, preserve the full sense of mutual self-giving and human procreation in the context of true love.' (*Gaudium et Spes,* n.51)

In the final editing of this text, there was an attempt to make 'the nature of the human person' and 'the nature of his acts' into two separate criteria. Those advocating this had a different understanding of natural law to that exemplified in the Fuchs quotation above. Their view would give the sexual act itself, quite independently of the person, its own intrinsic finality. This is a misunderstanding of the natural law, since it separates an action from the *person* performing it.

The sub-commission which prepared the final draft of *Gaudium et Spes* deliberately worded the above passage to make it quite clear that such an interpretation was not being accepted by Vatican II. While it rejected a purely subjectivist approach to morality (that is, one which only looked at a person's intentions and motives and which ignored the impact of what that person was actually doing), it made it quite clear that 'objective standards' included the person performing the action and did not refer simply to the act itself, considered as having a finality of its own independently of the person.

In opting for the more personalist interpretation of 'objective standards' the bishops at Vatican II certainly did not see themselves resolving the birth-control controversy in either direction. The Pope had explicitly reserved this matter to himself and he had set up his own Commission to advise him on it.

What the Council did was to leave the question open quite deliberately. This is clear from the way the drafting sub-commission handled both the text refered to above and also some last-minute 'modi' (i.e. suggested modifications) which were understood to have come from either the Pope himself or someone close to him. Shortly after Vatican II Professor Heylen, who was secretary of the Council's drafting sub-commission for this section of *Gaudium et Spes*, published a very thorough study of the passage from n.51 quoted on p.112 above. He states quite categorically that any translation or interpretation of *Gaudium et Spes* which would suggest that the teaching of Pius XI and Pius XII on artificial contraception 'is re-affirmed as certain and irreformable by the Council in no way corresponds to the real meaning of the text.' (*Ephemerides Theologicae Lovanienses*, 1966, p.564)

It was against this background that the papal birth-control Commission eventually presented their Report to the Pope. Their conclusion was that, given the right motivation and as long as the basic criteria outlined in *Gaudium et Spes* were respected, the Roman Catholic church would not be contradicting the natural law base of its fundamental teaching on marriage and the family, if it were to change its stance on the morality of artificial contraception. The Commission developed its line of argument at great length (full text in Harris, 1968, pp.216-244). At the risk of over-simplifying their closely reasoned submission, their basic stand could be summarised as follows.

If the person is an essential element in any objective evaluation of an action, the significance of the sexual act should not be deduced exclusively from the intrinsic working of the sexual faculty and its acts. To truly understand the significance of the sexual act we must also take into consideration the persons involved in that act. In more simple language, this means that the objective significance of an act of sexual intercourse between a couple cannot be understood in isolation from their relationship as persons and from the role that this act is playing within their relationship.

An act of sexual intercourse, therefore, which might be described as 'contraceptive' seen from the partial standpoint of the intrinsic working of the sexual faculty, could from a *human* standpoint (and that is what objective moral evaluation really means) be described as 'life-giving'. This is because such an act, seen in the personal context of this couple's relationship, could be 'life-giving' not only in the sense of sustaining and strengthening the life and love of the couple themselves but also in the sense of giving life to children as well. This follows from the fact that the well-being and consolidation of the loving relationship of the parents is an essential element in creating a home-base of security and acceptance which is so necessary for the children themselves if they are to be brought fully alive as persons secure enough to venture out to give and receive love. Such a climate of love and acceptance at home is one of the most crucial factors in the whole life-giving process. It is an integral part of what a married couple commit themselves to in their shared mission of giving fullness of life to their children by helping them to come alive as loving persons. Therefore, what from a partial viewpoint might be described as 'contraceptive' sexual intercourse, can more truly and more objectively be described as 'life-giving'.

It would be misleading to imply that the above position is really to be found in *Gaudium et Spes*. Nevertheless, by adopting the stance it did on 'objective morality' and natural law, the Council deliberately left the birth-control question open. Consequently, it would be equally misleading to suggest that this position contradicts the teaching of *Gaudium et Spes*.

HUMANAE VITAE – DISAGREEMENT OVER 'LIMITS' TO HUMAN DOMINION

Restoring the human person to the heart of Christian morality enabled Vatican II to articulate a very rich theology of human sexuality and married love in Chapter 1 of Part II of *Gaudium et Spes*. The implications of this personalist approach to married love were further elaborated by Paul VI in the first half of his famous 1968 encyclical letter, *Humanae Vitae*. In the following section of that encyclical the Pope gave his decision on artificial birth-control, a decision which he regarded as being equally firmly based on the personalist approach. The key sentence is:

'To experience the gift of married love while respecting the laws of conception is to acknowledge that one is not the master of the sources of life but rather the minister of the design established by the Creator. Just as man does not have unlimited dominion over his body in general, so also, and with more particular reason, he has no such dominion over his specifically sexual faculties, for these are concerned by their very nature with the generation of life, of which God is the source.' (n.13)

The objection has been raised that here the Pope seems to be identifying God's will with the intrinsic working of the sexual faculty and its acts and that this does not do full justice to the way Vatican II had presented 'objective standards'. The Pope, on the other hand, would insist that he is not isolating the sexual faculty from the human person; rather he is still being true to the personalist approach since he is stressing the fact that as *persons* we receive ourselves as gift from God. Therefore, our dominion over ourselves is not total. Since we have not created ourselves, we must respect the personal selves we have received as gift from God. To fail to do that is to fail to accept our humanity. It is to abuse God's gift and in so doing we betray our humanity and become 'inhuman'. Probably all the Christian churches would be prepared to agree with the Pope up to this point. In their statement on IVF almost all of them stress that there are 'limits' to our dominion over ourselves.

For instance, the Church of England report, *Personal Origins*, states:

'We accept that there is a structure and order in nature. We should therefore be concerned for the protection of its proper integrity and the realisation of its positive possibilities. We are not free to do as we please. There is a good to be aimed at, and this is the good of nature itself, as destined by God for realisation at the proper time. In thinking about human dominion we have a responsibility to make explicit the structural limits which define it. . .' (n.56, ii)

Chapter V of *Choices in Childlessness* is even entitled 'Limits and Limitations' and is rich in human and Christian insights about the 'limits' within which life has to be lived. For example, after noting that our 'creative, caring use of God-given powers cannot properly be exercised without limits', it comments: 'Theologically, a recognition of limits takes us right into the heart of God, who for the sake of his creation accepts the most radical limits on himself.' (p.39) For its part, the Evidence submitted to the Warnock Committee by the Baptist Union of Great Britain and Ireland states: 'There can be no absolute and fixed "processes of nature" which man must simply observe and not modify. The question is not a simple one, but the complex issue of finding where the limits are to man's co-creative work as a creature.' (p.4)

The key question, therefore, is not *whether* there are limits to humanity's dominion but rather *what* are these limits and how do we come to discern them. The parting of the ways for the churches comes when Pope Paul identifies the integrity of the exercise of the sexual faculty as a God-given limit. Once we interfere with the integrity of that faculty, he argues, we have gone beyond the limit. This is because such interference is tantamount to altering our very being as persons, and that is implicitly claiming that we can improve on the God-given gift of our humanity.

THE ROLE AND DEMANDS OF HUMAN REASON

Determining the limits to our dominion over nature is a task of human discernment. In a sense where we find the 'limit' is in our minds and our hearts — what Aquinas would call '*recta ratio*' (right-intentioned reason). We can never go beyond what we recognise to be 'reasonable', that is, in line with what we discern to be the true meaning of human life. And in determining what is 'reasonable', we must obviously grow in self-knowledge, both as individuals and as human race in general. This quest for true self-knowledge is at the heart of the story of human history, despite all its ups and downs. Down through the ages human beings have been growing in understanding of themselves as physical, psychological, emotional, sexual, relational, communicative, social and political beings. While this growth in knowledge does not imply a corresponding growth in human 'wisdom' (i.e. how we best use our knowledge to the benefit of humankind), it does mean that our understanding of 'being human' is constantly increasing and even changing. While admitting that God's image in us is marred, *Choices in Childlessness* says: 'God has given us the curiosity, inventiveness and power which move us to transcend given limits and limitations in order to create, under him, a new and better world.' (p.39)

Gaudium et Spes recognises this process going on and states quite frankly that God's Spirit is present within it. (n.26) This is not a surprising assertion if one accepts that the very heart of the natural law is nothing other than our 'right-intentioned reason' (*recta ratio*). After all, as Christians we believe that it is precisely into our minds and hearts that God's Spirit has been poured. And Aquinas does not hesitate to say that the essence of the New Law is 'the grace of the Holy Spirit revealing itself in faith working through love'. (*Summa Theologica*, I-II, 108, 1, corp.) This is echoed in the profound description of conscience found in *Gaudium et Spes:*

> 'Conscience is the most secret core and sanctuary of a man. There he is alone with God, whose voice echoes in his depths. In a wonderful manner conscience reveals that law which is fulfilled by love of God and neighbour. In fidelity to conscience, Christians are joined with the rest of men in the search for truth, and for the genuine solution to the numerous problems which arise in the life of individuals and from social relationships.' (n.16)

Of themselves the intrinsic structures of our human faculties do not tell us where the 'limit' to our human dominion lies. That is the task of human reflection, trying to discern which developments make us more human and which diminish our humanity and even lead us in the direction of inhumanity. Obviously, the intrinsic structures of our human faculties are part of the data to be considered in this reflective work of discernment. The above passage from *Gaudium et Spes* implies that this discernment process is part of a shared 'search for truth'. That is why dialogue is such an important part of the process.

WHAT IS 'PROPHETIC' ABOUT *HUMANAE VITAE*

It is no secret that many Roman Catholics, including many moral theologians, felt unable to accept the Pope's teaching on this matter. In fact, in the wake of *Humanae Vitae* many hierarchies throughout the world issued pastoral guide-lines to help Catholics come to terms with the encyclical. Some of these guide-lines offered reassurance to those who conscientiously could not accept the Pope's teaching. In the words of the Canadian bishops, such Catholics 'should not be considered, or consider themselves, shut off from the body of the faithful'. (Horgan, 1972, p.79) In a later statement (1/12/73) on the general theme of conscience, the Canadian bishops stressed that the presumption must always be in favour of the magisterium. However, as McCormick has pointed out, although such a presumption is essential to the 'Catholic context' of conscience and cannot be denied without denying the authority itself, nevertheless, it is still only a starting-point and of itself does not rule out the possibility of dissent. (cf. *The Search for Truth in the Catholic Context*, in *America*, 8/11/86, pp.276-281)

Seventeen years have elapsed since the publication of *Humanae Vitae*. In those years its teaching has been frequently reaffirmed by the hierarchical magisterium, most notably in the Apostolic Exhortation, *Familiaris*

Consortio, issued by John Paul II after the 1980 Synod. Yet the theological arguments have not been resolved. The basic question remains: why is the integrity of our use of our sexual faculties the limit to our God-given dominion over our human nature?

If the Roman Catholic position is substantially true, what lies at the heart of that truth needs to be teased out so that people can not only understand it but also appreciate its human goodness. In fact, the 1980 Synod made a plea for this. If the Roman Catholic position is touching on an important truth that is in danger of being overlooked but which at present is eluding all attempts to express it adequately, then our service to the truth demands that we continue to wrestle with whatever this position is trying to get at. And the same applies if there are important aspects of the truth which the Roman Catholic position has not yet taken fully aboard. There is no doubt that all three of these scenarios would benefit from ecumenical dialogue on this issue. Because of its importance both in itself and for its implications for IVF and for issues related to sexual ethics, I do not see how it could be left off the agenda. Maybe the new questions raised by IVF might help the churches to approach this well-worn issue with fresher and more receptive minds.

At the 1980 Synod in Rome some of the bishops spoke of the 'prophetic character' of *Humanae Vitae*. It could perhaps be argued that the 'prophetic' element in Paul VI's position lay in his insistence that we must not lose sight of the central importance of the sexual act in the language of life-giving love within marriage. If one grants a certain 'prophetic character' to his teaching in the sense just explained, perhaps one should also be willing to grant a similar 'prophetic character' in the teaching of some of the other churches too. Maybe the core insight Paul VI was struggling to preserve and articulate would have been better proclaimed, not as a moral absolute, but more along the lines of — 'treat the sexual act with reverence since here you are dealing with a reality which affects very deeply and intimately humankind's capacity for loving and giving life — and remember that life-giving love lies at the very heart of our being made in the image of God'.

As well as offering a more 'human' approach to birth control, interpreting Paul VI's 'prophetic' insight in this way might help to maintain a healthy respect and reverence for the normal human way of conceiving and giving birth to new life. This keeps the focus on the 'life-giving love' of the parents, without foreclosing any exploration of how that life-giving love can best be helped to bear fruit in children for couples whose marriage is infertile. Nor, on the other hand, would it rule out without further discussion the possibility of some married couples deliberately choosing to make their love 'life-giving' in ways other than by having children.

However, I must not anticipate the task of the inter-church dialogue. Certainly, exploring whether there could be a mutual enrichment of complementary insights leading to a common mind among the churches would surely be a major concern for any inter-church dialogue in this field.

THIRD QUESTION
'A grave sin to dare to risk murder' — does 'safety first' outweigh the claims of truth?

The 1974 *Declaration on Procured Abortion* from the Sacred Congregation for the Doctrine of the Faith stated: 'From a moral point of view this is certain: even if a doubt existed concerning whether the fruit of conception is already a human person, it is objectively a grave sin to dare to risk murder.' (n.13) Moreover, it backed up this assertion with a long footnote which needs careful examination:

> 'This declaration expressly leaves aside the question of the moment when the spiritual soul is infused. There is not a unanimous tradition on this point and authors are as yet in disagreement. For some it dates from the first instant, for others it could not at least precede nidation. It is not within the competence of science to decide between these views, because the existence of an immortal soul is not a question in its field. It is a philosophical problem from which our moral affirmation remains independent for two reasons: (1) supposing a later animation, there is still nothing less than a *human* life, preparing for and calling for a soul in which the nature received from parents is completed; (2) on the other hand it suffices that this presence of the soul be probable (and one can never prove the contrary) in order that the taking of life involve accepting the risk of killing a man, not only waiting for, but already in possession of his soul.' (footnote 19)

The validity of this 'safety first' line of argument needs to be looked at.

INTERPRETATION AND DECISION-MAKING

In making our judgments, empirical evidence has its rightful place. In popular parlance this part of the judgmental process is usually referred to as 'getting to know the facts'. This is what all the churches are doing when, in trying to arrive at a judgment about the status of the embryo, they examine the genetic and embryological evidence. This evidence is there for them all to see; at that level the 'facts' are clear, even though the empirical sciences are frequently discovering new evidence. Nevertheless, the churches all agree that empirical evidence alone is not sufficient. The 'facts' need to be interpreted in order to discover their human and moral significance. The Vatican Declaration has stressed this point: 'It is not up to biological sciences to make a definitive judgment on questions which are properly philosophical and moral, such as the moment when a human person is constituted or the legitimacy of abortion.' (n.13)

There is no dispute regarding the 'facts' about the embryo. The genetic and embryological evidence is perfectly clear and is laid out more or less fully in the position-statements of all the churches. What is doubtful, or at least disputed, is how this evidence is to be *interpreted*. Interpretation, however, is a judgment of evaluation. Therefore, although, as the Vatican Declaration admits, absolute certainty is unattainable in such a judgment, yet neither is it necessary. Interpretation operates in the field of moral certainty. That is the most it can claim for its judgments because it is the most that is open to us as human beings. But moral certainty is sufficient for us to act on. Therefore, when one has reached moral certainty regarding one's interpretation of the facts, one has every right to say, 'I am certain that this is true. And if I am to live in accordance with the truth, I must act in accordance with this certainty.'

In fact, the Roman Catholic church is able to accept this position when it comes to the other end of the life-cycle, the time of death. Some kind of criteria for ascertaining that death has occurred have to be accepted by the medical and legal professions and by society at large. The dying process has to be 'interpreted' by us. After a certain stage is reached, a judgment is made that a person is dead. This judgment is based on criteria drawn up by the medical profession. They have 'interpreted' the dying process *to the best of their knowledge*. They can feel morally certain that their criteria provide an adequate basis for responsible human action. However, absolute certainty is unattainable. New facts may come to light which might make them re-assess their medical definition of death. Human dying, like human coming-to-be, is more than a simple scientific fact. On this issue, even though the criteria for determining the moment of death have been a matter of considerable debate among doctors, the Roman Catholic church has left the judgment to the medical profession and has not insisted that they follow a 'safety first' approach in making their judgment. In fact, the Roman Catholic emphasis here has tended to be critical of an exaggerated 'safety first' approach insisted on by some doctors in caring for the terminally ill. Pius XII declared in 1957: 'It is in the physician's domain. . . to give a clear and precise definition of "death" and of the "moment of death" of a patient who dies without regaining consciousness . . . As to the pronouncement of death in certain particular cases, the answer cannot be inferred from religious and moral principles, and consequently, it is an aspect lying outside the competence of the Church.' (cf. *Acta Apostolicae Sedis,* vol 45, pp.1027-1033). There is no attempt to call on the 'safety first' argument on this issue.

Whenever we have the responsibility for making decisions which affect at a very deep level the good of other people, we have to have the confidence to act on our human judgments as long as they are made to the best of our ability. That kind of healthy attitude to decision-making is clearly present in the Roman Catholic church's teaching that we are not obliged to use extraordinary means to keep a person alive. In effect, this is saying that we can let our loved ones die in peace; we do not have to *prolong* their dying process. In certain circumstances, this can mean that we should have the confidence to let a loved one die when we actually have it in our power to keep that person alive for a while longer. Without suggesting that the two situations are parallel, at least it can be argued that a similar kind of confidence can be called for in decisions about the beginning of life. It is not sufficient to say: we can never have absolute certainty about the status of the embryo, so we must always treat it as a full human being, regardless of the consequences to others about whose full humanity we are in no doubt. The 'safety first' factor is only one element to be weighed up against other important values that might be involved. Karl Rahner is clearly assuming this to be the case when he considers the highly emotive and explosive issue of experimentation on human embryos:

'Catholic theology presupposes that at the moment of union of the male and female cells a *human being* comes into existence as an individual person with his own rights. *If* this is the case, such a person is no more an inconsequential passive object for experiments than the prisoners of Nazi concentration camps were. . . A one-hour-old human being has as much right to the integrity of his person as a human being of nine months or sixty years.

Nowadays, however, the above-mentioned presupposition is no longer held with certainty, but is exposed to positive doubt. . . Of course it does not follow from the fact of such an uncertainty that experiments with fertilised embryonic material are equivalent to morally indifferent experiments with mere "things". But it would be conceivable that, given a serious positive doubt about the human quality of the experimental material, the reasons in favour of experimenting might carry more weight, considered rationally, than the uncertain rights of a human being whose very existence is in doubt.' *Theological Investigations*, IX, p.236.

In conclusion, therefore, it must be said that, although the 'safety first' approach has much to commend it when what might be at risk is something as precious as human life, nevertheless its limitations need to be acknowledged since sometimes it is certain (and not just possible) that other fundamental human values are also involved.

FOURTH QUESTION

Could causing the death of an embryo ever be an expression of reverence for life?

Anyone who believes in reverence for life would instinctively answer 'no' to that question. In itself causing the death of an embryo is destroying life, not reverencing life. However, what the question is really asking is whether, in some circumstances, an action which includes bringing about the death of an embryo could be an action whose *fundamental human significance* is in keeping with reverence for life.

If the question is re-phrased in that way, the Roman Catholic position would be prepared to give an affirmative answer, since it accepts the legitimacy of what it calls 'indirect abortion' even though that involves causing the death of an embryo. An indirect abortion is an abortion which comes about as an unavoidable by-product of an action which has some other purpose quite independent of the abortion and which would still achieve this purpose even if the mother were not pregnant.

Many moral theologians are unhappy about the notion of 'indirect' abortion as traditionally explained. It seems to play havoc with our normal way of looking at our responsibility for our actions. If I set an action in motion which I know full well will result in a certain thing happening, I am responsible for what happens as a result of my action. Maybe I would prefer it not to happen. Yet I know it will certainly happen and, despite that certain knowledge, I still perform the action which will bring it about. It would seem more satisfactory to say that we must accept responsibility for the bad elements in our actions as well as for their good elements. To perform an action which has some element of evil involved in it would usually be regarded as justified, provided that the good which is also involved is substantial enough to outweigh the evil.

This is not the same as saying that the end justifies the means. That principle could justify all manner of inhuman action. 'The end justifies the means' is completely unacceptable and totally inadequate as a moral principle.

Nevertheless, the end for which an action is performed is very relevant to the moral evaluation of that action. Traditionally, Roman Catholic moral theology has spoken of three factors to be considered in the moral evaluation of any action — the object (i.e. the action being done — not an easy thing to determine because of the close link between an action and its consequences!), the intention and the circumstances. Until these three factors are considered together, we have not yet reached a proper 'moral' evaluation of an action. We are still at a 'pre-moral' stage. That is why, if causing the death of an embryo is involved in the action under consideration, some writers would refer to it as a 'pre-moral' evil at this stage of the evaluation process. Causing the death of an embryo in itself is evil; there is nothing positively good about it. It is destroying life. However, in the apparently very rare instance when the existence of the embryo within the mother is a very real threat to her life, there is an additional morally relevant factor which needs to be considered in coming to a moral evaluation of the action.

Those involved in this action, prior to their deciding whether it is morally good or not (therefore, still at the 'pre-moral' stage), see that the action has a good and a bad side to it. It will kill the embryo (the evil side of the action) and it will remove what is threatening the life of the mother (the good side). Until these two sides of the action are weighed up and a moral decision is made, they can appropriately be referred to as the 'pre-moral evil' and the 'pre-moral good' involved in the action which is being contemplated. When the moral decision is made, it embraces the whole action with its amalgam of good and evil. It can be interpreted as 'morally good' if the good involved is of sufficient weight to offset the evil involved in the action. The true 'moral' description of such an action will be in terms of the good it brings about. This is the predominant 'meaning' of the action. Thus, an abortion which removes an embryo threatening the life of the mother can rightly and more appropriately be termed a 'life-saving' action in terms of its moral significance.

Why this analysis differs from the unacceptable 'end justifies the means' approach is that there one is not dealing with an action having *within it* different elements which need to be weighed up in order to arrive at a moral evaluation of the action as a whole. The objection against the 'end justifies the means' approach is that it can be used to justify an action which is entirely or predominantly evil in itself and which does not have *within it* any good elements of sufficient weight to off-set the evil involved. The action in question merely creates a situation in which some good effect either can or does follow by way of a quite distinct human action (e.g. the good intended through taking hostages, threatening reprisals, torturing a suspect etc).

The kind of analysis I have been describing is very different. It is by means of this kind of analysis that many people who believe that the status of the embryo should be interpreted in the strongest sense ('full human dignity') are able to reconcile this belief with the possibility of abortion for a sufficiently grave reason — and saving the life of the mother is accepted as such a grave reason. It is precisely their reverence for life, that basic good of the human person, which in this instance enables them to face up to the tragedy that both lives cannot be saved and so everything possible must be done to save one. Reverence for life, therefore, is the dominant meaning of this action which includes within it abortion as one of its constituent elements. In other words, *what from one angle might be described as an abortion, from another angle could be described as a life-saving action.* Saving the life of the mother is normally regarded as the only reason sufficiently grave to justify an abortion in this way; however, some Roman Catholic moral theologians, especially in the United States, are raising the possibility of other grave reasons as well. (cf. Lotstra 1985, pp.128-130)

If Christians who hold the 'full respect' position are able to accept the possibility that, in certain circumstances, an action which involves causing the death of the embryo can still truly be regarded as a life-reverencing action, it is not surprising that this also holds true for those Christians who do not interpret the embryo as having the full dignity of a human being. For those who think in this way, reverence for the life of a human being will mean that their prime focus is on the mother — and, to a lesser extent, on the other human beings involved, the father, the rest of the family, etc. Although they accept that reverence is due to the embryo, they still do not see it as having the full dignity of a human being. Hence, they will necessarily interpret respect for human life and the human person primarily in terms of the life of the mother and those whose lives are linked to hers at a very intimate level. Therefore, when the life, or health, or substantial well-being of the mother is in tragic conflict with the continued existence of the embryo, for those who follow this position it would be a denial of the full reverence owed to the mother to sacrifice her substantial good for the sake of the less-than-full reverence due to the embryo. According to this way of thinking, causing the death of the embryo in such a case would once again be seen as one element in a human action which substantially should be interpreted as an act of reverence for human life and the human person. In fact, refraining from such an action would, in this view, be interpreted as a violation of respect for human life and the human person.

Some people who think in this way prefer to use the expression 'termination of pregnancy' on the grounds that the termination of the pregnancy and the death of the embryo are distinct realities, even though they are *de facto* inseparable at present.

FIFTH QUESTION

What about evidence which points in a contrary direction and suggests that fertilisation is not the key moment in determining the status of the embryo?

THE 'GIFT' OF CONTRARY EVIDENCE

It has been stated above that all the Christian churches recognise the need to listen to all the evidence of modern genetics and embryology. Of itself this evidence will not solve the philosophical question of the status of the human embryo. Nevertheless, it is the scientific evidence that has to be interpreted by the churches and by philosophers. Moreover, none of the evidence can be ignored. That is why we must be careful not to ignore 'contrary' evidence — evidence that makes us question our interpretation. To wrestle with the problem of 'contrary' evidence can open out new paths to us in the search for truth. Karl Popper even goes so far as to say that we should actually welcome empirical evidence which demonstrates the falsity of our original hypothesis, however dear that hypothesis might be to us. Such 'contrary' evidence can stimulate us to elaborate a more comprehensive hypothesis and so can enable us to get closer to the truth of things. I treasure Bryan Magee's comment on Popper's position: 'The man who welcomes and acts on criticism will prize it almost above friendship: the man who fights it out of concern to maintain his position is clinging to non-growth.' (Bryan Magee, *Popper*, Fontana, 1973, p.39)

As a Roman Catholic I feel it is important, therefore, to take note of any scientific facts which would seem to constitute 'contrary evidence' to the position that fertilisation is the key moment, after which the embryo must be accorded full human respect. Two such pieces of contrary evidence are frequently mentioned.

The first is the possibility of twinning and even of consequent recombination during the first few weeks. It seems that the possibility of twinning actually occurring is statistically very small. However, it also appears to be the case that it would be at least theoretically possible by human intervention to make it happen in every fertilised ovum. This puts a large question-mark against the claim that we are dealing with a human individual at this early stage, since the stage of definitive individuation has not yet been reached. Without definitive individuality it seems impossible philosophically to speak of a human being in the proper sense of the word. I am informed that recent embryological research is finding some evidence that the phenomenon of twinning might have its origin in the very beginnings of cell-duplication. Depending on the exact nature of this evidence, it might be possible that, if substantiated, it would provide an empirical basis for claiming definitive individuality for twins from the first moment of cell-duplication. However, that would hardly be the case if recombination remained a possibility, even if only by artificial means. Moreover, it is not clear what such evidence would mean for the possibility of artificially causing twinning in any embryo during the first fourteen days. If that still seemed to be possible, the question-mark against definitive individuation would still seem to remain.

The other piece of 'contrary evidence' is the phenomenon of foetal wastage. It appears that a large number of fertilised ova never actually implant in the mother's womb; and that, of those which do implant, a significant number are lost in the course of the pregnancy. The precise figure for wastage prior to implantation does not seem to be universally agreed by the medical profession. Some have claimed it to be as high as 70%. On the other hand, it is claimed that some new evidence is coming to light which suggests that it might be as low as 8%. Even if this latter figure proves to be correct, it does not eliminate the phenomenon and the questions it raises.

Some people would claim that it raises no questions at all. After all, they would say, natural disasters are part of human life. No one would claim that that fact gives us the right to imitate such natural disasters and destroy life ourselves. Obviously that is perfectly true. However, those who argue in this way are overlooking the fact that natural disasters really are *disasters*. Human ingenuity usually leaves no stone unturned to try to prevent natural disasters occurring. In fact, it would be regarded as a heinous crime if people had the ability to avert a massive natural disaster and yet did nothing about it. They would be condemned as guilty of culpable neglect. There seems to be no evidence of a similar reaction to the so-called natural disaster of foetal wastage. I do not get the impression that even the most committed 'anti-abortion' doctors would adopt that approach to foetal wastage. They and their medical colleagues do not consider the prevention of foetal wastage to be a high medical priority. In fact, far from seeing it as a priority, I suspect that the medical profession would view the elimination of foetal wastage as undesirable. The medical profession seems to interpret the phenomenon as a kind of natural selection process whereby embryos which are defective in some way fail to proceed to full term.

The question-mark against the full humanity of the embryo, therefore, does not come directly from the phenomenon of foetal wastage itself but from what seems to be a universal reaction to this phenomenon. The fact that foetal wastage is accepted as a desirable and beneficial phenomenon suggests that the death of the embryo in this instance is not interpreted as any kind of human tragedy. That in turn seems to indicate that in this instance people in general do not seem to be reacting to the embryo as they would to a human being in the proper sense of the word.

THE COMMON ESTIMATION OF PEOPLE

The 'contrary evidence' in this second instance, therefore, is really based on what might be called 'the common estimation of people'. This might sound a very weak argument. In reality, it is a factor to which many philosophers pay very special attention. It is true, of course, that popular opinion can more easily be manipulated in these days of mass media; nor would one want to claim that morality can be reduced to the level of a majority vote. Yet, despite those caveats, the common estimation of people is not to be overlooked, especially when it concerns the interpretation of the more basic experiences of life itself. Even the idea of 'reading the signs of the times', to which Vatican II gave such importance, is related to the notion of the common estimation of people.

That is why it is useful to think about the standing of the embryo in the common estimation of people. Admittedly, it is impossible to get to know with complete accuracy what is the common estimation of people on an issue such as the status of the embryo. Nevertheless, I would dare to suggest that Lotstra is not too far off the mark when he describes what he believes to be the common mind of very many people:

> 'They do not recognise the foetus as a full human being but neither will they have it treated as waste matter, and they definitely evaluate the termination of its existence in the light of the dignity of human life. At the same time they credit

the intervention (i.e. abortion) for the remedy it provides to the conditions of serious maternal or parental distress. The foetus, therefore, has a special status but abortion is deemed permissible in certain cases and up to a certain point of gestation.' (*Abortion: the Catholic Debate in America*, Irvington, New York, 1985, p.291)

All the churches agree that the scientific evidence needs *interpretation*. The most rudimentary level of this interpretation lies in the common estimation of people, even though this level of interpretation needs further refinement.

Language can be a helpful indicator of how we interpret reality. That is why it is interesting to note that we do not call a fertilised hen's egg a chicken or an acorn growing in the ground an oak tree. They are different realities. The fertilised egg is precisely what we say it is — a fertilised hen's egg. It will become a chicken in time but it is not yet one. It has the potential to become a chicken. Scholastic philosophy might also say that it is a chicken in *potency* but it would not say that it is *actually* a chicken. Ransil applies the same line of thinking to the early stages of human development: 'No one looking at the zygote and its immediate successive forms will equate them with a human being, just as he will not call a fertilised hen's egg a chicken.' (cf. Lotstra 1985, p.111) He is suggesting that the zygote, the embryo and the 5-month-old foetus are also just what we say they are — a zygote, an embryo and a 5-month-old foetus. They are necessary stages in the development of a human being in the full sense of the word. Therefore they must be treated with reverence. But the reverence they are to be given is no more and no less than the reverence due to a zygote, an embryo and a 5-month-old foetus. It is not the reverence to be given to a viable foetus or to a new-born baby or to the mother herself.

It would be interesting to explore whether this line of interpretation is confirmed by the way women who are pregnant speak about what is going on within them. Does there come a time when a woman changes from referring to herself as pregnant and starts speaking *in the present tense* about the 'baby'? If so, it would perhaps give an indication of the way she is interpreting the reality within her. Maybe that is why our forebears considered 'quickening' to be a significant moment in the development of a human being, though probably the impact of 'quickening' has been overtaken today by the experience both parents are able to share of seeing their 'baby' on the scanner. This line of thought is not suggesting that the dignity of the human embryo depends on the attitude of the mother towards it. None of the churches would accept such a subjective criterion. As we have seen already, they all insist that the dignity of the embryo is 'recognised' by us; it is not 'conferred' by us.

Nevertheless, the mother's perception is not without significance. In a sense, it is 'human interpretation' at its most basic level. The mother might not be a professional philosopher but how she and millions of mothers like her 'interpret' the human experience of pregnancy might be some indicator of what is really happening. A further indicator might be the different impact of a miscarriage on a woman depending on how far on in the pregnancy it occurs. This approach is obviously very tentative. Its validity would need to be tested by some empirical research on how women actually experience their pregnancy. It could even happen, of course, that such research might point in the opposite direction and provide an additional reason for interpreting the human embryo as fully human from the very moment of fertilisation.

EXTENDING THE DIALOGUE

Some Christian churches, though sympathetic to the strong Roman Catholic stance against abortion, are put off by the absoluteness of that stance. They feel they could join a united front with the Roman Catholic church on this issue if the latter's position was a little more nuanced. Perhaps a re-examination of the 'safety first' argument might provide some kind of opening in this direction. It is certainly true that some Roman Catholic moral theologians are already arguing for a more nuanced position and are raising questions about the full humanity of the embryo in the earliest stages following conception.

For instance, John Mahoney, undoubtedly the most respected Roman Catholic moral theologian in Britain, explores some of the implications of footnote 19 of the Vatican Declaration (cf. p.119 above):

> 'What the (Vatican) Declaration does not assert is that this living being is a human person (it deliberately. . . leaves this question open). The most it appears to claim is that it "probably" is, since the contrary can never be proved. To entertain, however, even the possibility that there can be for a period of time a living human being, or a living human entity, which does not possess a human soul and is not therefore a human person, is a major concession, which, however, raises many questions concerning the status of this non-ensouled, non-personal, human entity. It cannot, for one thing, have any rights, since traditional Catholic doctrine holds that rights flow from the status of being a person. It appears, in fact, to be none other than human tissue. It is undoubtedly alive; it is clearly of human origin; and it is genetically unique, both as human and as

individually human, in the sense that there is none other like it. Given appropriate favourable circumstances for development, of course, it will, in due time, develop into an "ensouled" being and therefore a human person . . . It may well be that the status of this living being on the way to hominisation is comparable in significant ways to the status of primates (to go back no further) at a prehuman stage in the evolution of *homo sapiens*, as we now identify that evolutionary process.' (*Bioethics and Belief*, p.82)

Against that background and in the light of his earlier detailed analysis of the congregation's arguments, Mahoney eventually reaches the following challenging conclusion:

'. . . the most one can conclude of the 'probability' that ensoulment occurs at conception is that it is possible but, when all is taken into account, rather unlikely. What then becomes of the ethical consequences deriving from the status of the fertilised ovum and the embryo in its early stages of development? And to what degree would one who destroyed such a being be incurring the risk of committing homicide, as the Vatican Declaration asserts? There is no doubt, of course, that one would be destroying something which is alive, but the question is, is it more than live human tissue? The degree of moral risk corresponds to the degree of likelihood that what one is dealing with is an ensouled human person. Accordingly, if one considers it just possible, but quite unlikely, that one is faced with a human person, the risk that in destroying it one is deliberately killing or destroying such a person must be considered correspondingly slight.' (pp.82-83)

Of course Mahoney is speaking only of the early embryo, since he subscribes to the 'full respect' position once the embryo has achieved definitive individuation. However, he is prepared to examine the possible practical conclusions of the position he has been exploring. For instance, he suggests that reasons sufficiently serious to justify someone deciding to destroy the early embryo might be those 'affecting either that being's own prospects for the future, as in cases of genetic abnormality, or the life and welfare of others, as in cases of rape and incapacity in a woman to carry a child to term without risk to herself.' (p.85) Later in the book, in a paragraph which he insists is 'of a markedly tentative nature' (p.98), Mahoney suggests that, 'given a sufficient reason', embryo experimentation (involving the inevitable death of the embryo) might also qualify as truly respectful.

In fact, Mahoney is far from being the only Roman Catholic moral theologian to express reservations about the Roman Catholic position. Hans Lotstra has studied the debate on abortion among Catholics in the U.S.A.

in recent years, *Abortion: The Catholic Debate in America,* (Irvington, New York, 1985). One of his conclusions is: 'The majority of American Catholic moralists do have reservations about the Church's declared stand on abortion.' (p.275) Furthermore, he adds in a footnote: 'In other parts of the world also there has been growing diversity on abortion among Catholic moralists.' (footnote 2, p.299)

As yet, the Christian churches have not been able to arrive at a mutually agreed interpretation of the status of the embryo. The problem some people have with the position which argues for the full humanity of the embryo is not its profound respect for the embryo from its earliest moment of existence. They can warm to that respect and feel in tune with it. Where they part company is in its claim that that respect or reverence is on exactly the same level as the reverence to be given to a human being in the full sense of the word. That does not tune in with the reverence they instinctively feel towards the embryo in its early stages of development. And the problem other people have with the more 'permissive' positions is not the care and concern they express for the mother and the other members of the family who might be involved. That care and concern strikes a sympathetic chord with them. Where they are dissatisfied with these more 'permissive' positions is that, despite their protestations of reverence and respect for the embryo from its earliest moments, it is hard to see how this reverence and respect is to be cashed in the hard currency of decision-making in conflict situations. Their instinctive feeling towards the embryo in its early stages of development demands more than the mere rhetoric of reverence and respect.

Therefore, together the Christian churches need to continue the search for a more satisfactory interpretation of the evidence. It could be that we still have something to learn from the instinctive 'gradualism' of our Christian forebears over many centuries. Although they viewed the abortion of the 'unformed' foetus as not equivalent to homicide and as a sin of lesser gravity than abortion of the 'formed' foetus, yet they still looked on it as a serious evil since it involved the destruction of life that was human in some way at least. Of course, their 'gradualism' would need to be unpacked in terms which make sense to us today. In looking again at their instinctive interpretation of abortion, we might also need to disentangle it from their very defective knowledge of the processes of human generation and from some of the philosophical influences which marred their full appreciation of the goodness of human sexuality. The aim of dialogue among the Christian churches on this issue would be to arrive at an interpretation which did full justice to all the evidence and which would provide some kind of acceptable criterion which would help people to give proper reverence both to the embryo and to the mother and her family.

Conclusion

In this chapter I have tried to be self-critical as a Roman Catholic. It is possible that what I have written will provoke a reaction from other Roman Catholics. That is a risk worth taking, provided that this chapter also provokes Christians in the other churches to be similarly self-critical in an open way about their own position. However, this chapter will be counter-productive if it merely focuses attention on the Roman Catholic question-marks I have high-lighted without any similar airing of possible deficiencies in the positions adopted by the other churches.

7

Directions and difficulties in ecumenical dialogue

In its deepest sense reverence for life is not a moral attitude which a person adopts by free choice. It is a human reaction in the face of the wonder of life. It is, therefore, dependent on a person's capacity actually to see and appreciate the wonder of life. Such a capacity is not reliant on or in proportion to education in the formal sense of the word. Rather it demands a kind of purity or simplicity of vision, a vision which has not been blinded by a person's having become captivated by all sorts of lesser attractions which have monopolised his or her attention.

In this sense, reverence before life is a religious experience. It is becoming conscious of our finitude in the face of life. It makes us aware of our dependence, our limitations and ultimately of our mortality. But this awareness is not born of self-depreciation but of wonder in the face of the immensity, all-pervasiveness and continuity of life. I cannot truly reverence life and at the same time act as though I am the centre of the universe. Reverence for life is not a solitary or isolating experience. It is a consciousness of belonging, of being part of something much greater than myself.

Such reverence for life is not exclusive to Christians. Some might even say it is not even characteristic of Christians. Yet it is an essential element in genuine human religious experience. Without it our eyes are still closed to the wonder of God around us and within us. Without it a Christian might be 'practising' in the sense of 'attending church' but might still not be a 'believing' Christian, since he or she will not yet have become aware of the level of life at which we actually experience the reality of God.

Reverence before life is a gift, something given to us. In other words, reverence before life is dependent upon life being given in the first place. Reverence before life is part of the gift of being God's creature.

It is not abstract *idea* of life that elicits the movement of reverence within us. It is life itself as we encounter it within us and around us, in people and in the whole of God's creation. It is those experiences in which we seem to be in contact with life at a very deep level — the experiences of birth and death, of love and suffering, of hope and fear, of security and alienation. It is the way we encounter life in animals, in trees and flowers, in all the living organisms that make up our world. 'Life must go on' is a common expression. The advance of our scientific understanding today enables us to appreciate a new depth of meaning in that expression. Modern genetics and embryology have brought home to us just how true it is that life does go on. We human beings are part of the flow of life. Life went on before us, and it goes on all around us, and it will continue to go on after us. We are not visitors to life, calling in for a few decades from some extra-life domain, and then passing on elsewhere on our journey. We belong to life. Life has thrown us up and so life cannot disown us, even in our death. The life we have has been passed on to us and we in our turn pass it on to future generations.

All this might sound like a kind of animism. In fact, it is essentially very different from animism. Animism would identify this all-pervading and on-going life with God himself. Whereas the view of life given above interprets life in the light of the doctrine of creation which would say that life, all life, comes from God but is not to be identified with God. It is the handiwork of God through which we get a glimpse of the wonder of God himself, just as in a work of art we get a glimpse of the genius of the artist. The artist puts himself or herself into a work of art but remains distinct from it. God puts himself into creation but remains distinct from and other than creation. de Mello's 'Master' expresses this point well:

'Disciple: How does one seek union with God?
Master: The harder you seek, the more distance you create between Him and you.
Disciple: So what does one do about the distance?
Master: Understand that it isn't there.
Disciple: Does that mean that God and I are one?
Master: Not one. Not two.
Disciple: How is that possible?
Master: The sun and its light, the ocean and the wave, the singer and his song — not one. Not two.' (Anthony de Mello, *One Minute Wisdom*, Sujarat Sahitya Prakesh, Anand, India, 1985, p.34)

Without reverence for life our reverence for the human person is seriously deficient. To isolate the human person from the rest of creation is to see things with a distorted vision. It is no longer reverence in the full sense of the word. It can even become a form of idolatry, turning humanity into a god instead of seeing the human person as very much part of creation, while still being its crown. Human progress and fulfilment is an integral part of bringing creation to its fulfilment. The rest of creation is not simply a resource to be exploited arbitrarily by human beings in their quest for some kind of human perfection totally separate from the rest of creation. True human progress is the integrated progress of humanity within creation, rather than our standing over and against creation.

Reverence for life and the churches' discussion of IVF

What has reverence in this fundamental sense to do with the 'respect for life' we talk about when the issue of IVF comes up for discussion? As we have seen, Christian churches adopt different positions regarding the status of the embryo. These basic positions can lead to practical conclusions which may seem diametrically opposed to each other. The fundamental question is: do these differing churches all start from the same position of reverence for life and merely disagree on how reverence is to be expressed practically? Or does their difference go much deeper, with the implication that one or other position is tantamount to a denial of reverence for life.

All the Christian churches would claim that 'reverence for life' is a fundamental factor in their approach to God and his Creation. Because of that, they would naturally feel disturbed and affronted by any suggestion that they were actually aligning themselves with any 'anti-life' camp. They would experience a similar disturbance and affront if the churches which differed from them claimed the 'pro-life' label exclusively for themselves.

Christianity is a 'pro-life' faith

Christianity is essentially a 'pro-life' faith. To appreciate what this means, we need to identify what we mean by an 'anti-life' position.

Any position which denies that a human person, precisely as a human person, should be revered and respected is an 'anti-life' position. So too is a position which so exalts human beings that it isolates them totally from the rest of Creation and gives them the right to violate, desecrate and even destroy God's Creation simply to satisfy their arbitrary desires or in order to enhance their delusions of power. Throughout history positions which have claimed to be fundamentally 'pro-life' have been spoiled by 'anti-life' elements hidden within them. This has been evident even in Christianity itself.

Denying certain basic human rights to particular groups of people is a violation of reverence. Actually to take away their life is the highest form of irreverence. That is why such emphasis is laid on respect for *human life*. However, this immediately raises a further question. When we are talking about respect for *human life,* we are talking about respect for the *life of human persons.* However, as we have seen above, nowadays we are becoming more conscious of the continuity of human life as such and the complexity of this process of continuity. We are also becoming much more aware of how closely human life is linked to the other forms of life which make up creation. Therefore, an important question which is posed to us today and which cannot be evaded by the churches is: is it legitimate to draw a distinction between *human life* and the *life of a human person;* and, if so, is this distinction one of substantial moral significance?

This question is clearly of key importance when the kind of reverence owed to the human embryo is discussed. The Roman Catholic position would say that, for all practical purposes, from the moment of fertilisation the life of the human embryo is to be given the same reverence as the life of a human person. Hence, that position would not grant any moral significance to such a distinction, even if the distinction itself was accepted as legitimate. On the other hand, the positions of most of the other Christian churches would differ from the Roman Catholic position on this. While granting that the life of the embryo can truly be called 'human life', they would regard the embryo as calling for lesser reverence from us until it reached that stage when, according to the various criteria they suggest, it becomes a human being in the full and proper sense of the word. For them, therefore, there would be a real distinction between human life and the life of a human person (or human being in the full and proper sense of the word) and this distinction would be very significant from an ethical point of view. Further consideration of this important question must be left to the churches to undertake in their dialogue together.

Reverence for life compatible with disagreement about the embryo

If the climate of trust and mutual acceptance needed for genuine dialogue is to be present, those on opposite sides in the debate need to appreciate how those who differ from them can still have a very real reverence for human life.

The mystery of life elicits our reverence at the whole variety of levels where it makes its impact upon us. Perhaps true growth in holiness really means this sense of wonder before the mystery of life gradually extending into all the levels of our experience. The same would apply to the corresponding sense of horror and revulsion whenever there is a deliberate violation of that life before which we feel a sense of reverence. This sense of horror and revulsion is an essential element of our sense of reverence.

If we all lived at the level of achieved holiness or wholeness, our heightened level of awareness would leave us constantly moved both by deep reverence and wonder and also by horror and revulsion. Admittedly, even if we were living at such a level (if it were humanly possible), we would still have to accept our human limitations and recognise that we would not be able to respond through active involvement in working for all these good causes; our engagement would necessarily have to be selective.

Needless to say, we are not living at that level of fully achieved holiness or wholeness. We are all operating only at a partial level. That is why we can at one and the same time be both sensitive and insensitive to human life issues. We can be vividly aware at one level and quite blind at another level. This is not unlike the phenomenon from our human experience which is described very clearly by Gerard Hughes S.J.:

'. . . our minds have layers upon layers of consciousness. At one level of consciousness I may be full of faith that all power belongs to God and that without him I can do nothing. Then my security is threatened in some way and I reach a deeper level of consciousness to which my faith has not penetrated and where I have been living in a state of unconscious atheism. This moment of crisis is an invitation to grow in faith. Then another crisis occurs and I become aware of an even deeper level of atheism within me. In our journey towards God we proceed like those small birds whose flight is in loops. They always seem to be about to drop, but the drop in their flight seems to urge them forwards.' (*God of Surprises,* DLT, 1985, pp.100-101)

Perhaps something similar happens with regard to our sense of reverence — it may even be just another form of the same phenomenon. We can have a heightened sense of reverence for human life issues at one level and yet be quite blind to other human life issues at another level. And this might be true of us not just as individuals but also as Christian communities and churches.

If there is some truth in this, I would suggest two consequences which would seem to flow from it:
(1) If we are concentrating on very specific issues relating to reverence for human life, we should be careful about our choice of slogans or about the titles we give to our movements. If we are 'pro-life' at one layer of

our living, it could be that we are actually 'anti-life' at another layer. And those who are very strongly 'pro-life' at that second layer might well be experiencing us as 'anti-life' from their vantage point. And vice-versa: we in our turn might experience them as 'anti-life'.

(2) We must be particularly attentive to the criticisms of those who experience us as 'anti-life'. It could well be that they are the very people who can cure us of our blindness to our 'anti-life' dimension in this layer of life.

This notion of layers of reverence might have something to offer to the Christian churches in their dialogue about the status of the embryo. Our sense of reverence will probably be somewhat different for all of us depending on the differing experiences we have had. After all, the kind of 'reverence' we are considering here is not some abstract idea but a very profound movement of the human spirit. It will naturally tend to be greatest in those areas of life on which we have focused most of our attention. This will especially be the case if we have invested a great deal of commitment and love into promoting reverence for life in these areas.

For instance, people who have been deeply involved with issues concerning the plight of women in all kinds of situations of oppression or discrimination will naturally focus on the person of the mother and the effect that this unwanted pregnancy will have on her life. This natural focus will be still further magnified if the pregnancy in question is the result of an actual act of oppression against the woman — for instance, if she has been raped (even by her husband!) or if she is the victim of incestuous intercourse. Reverence for the life of the woman and a consequent desire to let her live her life in real freedom might be so central to the focus of such people that they might well find it incredible, in terms of reverence for life as they experience it, that others should want to oblige the woman to accept this pregnancy on the grounds that the same reverence is owed to an embryo as is owed to this woman. In such a case, they would interpret this demand as a further compounding of the oppression against the woman. Consequently, such a demand would fill them with horror and revulsion and they would react against it very strongly.

Such people would claim that they too are motivated by a genuinely 'pro-life' commitment. They are not saying that the woman should have an abortion. They are simply arguing that the reverence due to her means that she should be able to choose freely either to have her child or abort it. If she is denied the possibility of an abortion, they would argue, she is also denied the possibility of freely choosing to have her child. Even though many initially unwilling mothers make a virtue out of necessity and come to accept their child and are able to give it great love, this position would argue that this is second-best and might have within it the seeds of future psychological problems regarding personal relationships.

The same might be true of those who are deeply involved in problems of family care, especially in instances where another child can sometimes bring about the break-up of the whole family unit or at least the break-down of one or both of the parents and the consequent disastrous effects for the rest of the family. Reverence for the life of the family would be the driving inspiration of such people and so their tendency would be to make the good of the whole family the prime focus of their basic reverence before life. Seeing things from this angle, they might find themselves unable to believe that the same reverence is owed to an embryo as is owed to the persons who make up this whole family unit. Once again they would not be arguing for an abortion as an automatic solution; in fact, it might be no solution at all. They would merely be arguing that reverence for the family and for the persons making up the family should be the prime focal-point and so the possibility of an abortion should not be automatically ruled out.

Dialogue means really listening to the other person — and not just to the words uttered. Even more importantly it means listening to the feelings and experiences which can lie behind the words. Inter-church dialogue about the kind of reverence due to the embryo implies trying to think inside the minds and hearts of men and women who have a deep reverence for human life and who are committed to promoting the dignity of the human person and yet who may hold a very different position to one's own.

Our commitment to ecumenism, which John Paul II referred to in Liverpool as 'one of the main concerns of the Church in the last part of the twentieth century', obliges us to try to appreciate Christian moral stances which differ from our own and even to explore whether these positions might be emphasising aspects of the truth that we are underrating. Although ecumenism does not mean compromising on the truth or trying to establish some kind of lowest common denominator, yet basic inter-church disagreements on certain moral issues can lead us to wonder whether the way each of us sees and articulates the truth at present is really doing full justice to that truth. It is too easy to say: one of us must be wrong — and obviously it is not us! Maybe the fact that we differ should lead us to say: possibly none of us is completely right. That would not be compromising the truth. It would be respecting the truth and our need to be continually searching for a better understanding of it. Maybe one of our positions has more to be said for it than appears at first sight to the others. That is why we must really try to understand and appreciate what each other is trying to say. Maybe none of our positions are really adequate. That is why we must not turn our backs on exploring the possibility of some other interpretation of the facts which everyone might come to accept as the best current expression of the truth. Naturally, the importance of inter-church dialogue gives no justification for sloppy thinking or weak argumentation. Respectful listening to each other implies having the kindness and honesty to point out factual errors or invalid arguments when they occur — but that is a kindness one would want to have reciprocated too!

Some suggested rules for dialogue

For the remainder of this chapter I shall examine some suggestions that might help to make dialogue both possible and fruitful on the highly emotive question of the status of the embryo. They are rules for dialogue which were originally put forward in the context of the abortion debate. While they obviously apply to dialogue about the status of the embryo, since that is central to the abortion debate, they could be equally helpful for ecumenical dialogue on other issues of ethical concern.

Richard McCormick, a highly respected U.S. moral theologian, has outlined ten 'rules for conversation' for those who differ on the abortion issue, cf. *How Brave a New World?* (SCM, London, 1981) pp.176-188:

(1) *Attempt to identify areas of agreement.* Under the heading of this rule he makes the comment:

> 'Both those who find abortion morally repugnant and those who do not would agree that abortion is, in most cases, a tragic thing, an undesirable thing . . . Therefore, all discussants should be clear-headedly and wholeheartedly behind policies that attempt to frustrate the personal and social causes of abortion.' (p.177)

(2) *Avoid the use of slogans.* He mentions two slogans which he regards as unjustified. One is the use of the term 'murder' to describe abortion. He comments:

> '"Murder" is a composite value term that means (morally) unjustified killing of another person . . . To use that term does not clarify an argument if the very issue at stake is justifiability. Rather it brands a position and, incidentally, those who hold it. It is a conversation stopper.' (p.178)

The other slogan he would outlaw from the conversation is 'a woman has a right to her own body'. He describes this slogan as 'the conclusion of an often unexamined argument and therefore a slogan with some questionable assumptions'. Among such questionable assumptions he lists: 'that the foetus is, for these purposes, a part of the woman's body; that rights over one's body are absolute; that abortion has nothing to do with a husband.' (p.178)

(3) *Represent the opposing position accurately and fairly.*

(4) *Distinguish the pairs right-wrong, good-bad.* According to McCormick, the right-wrong pair refers to the intrinsic quality of the action done, prescinding from the subjective state of the person doing the action. The good-bad pair refers to the intention or motivation of the person doing the action and prescinds from the intrinsic quality of the action itself. McCormick, therefore, is stressing the importance of making a clear distinction between a person's intention or motivation and the actual rightness or wrongness of the act in itself. From the best of intentions and motivated by the highest ideals a person might mistakenly perform an action which is wrong in itself and thus bring about harm. Conversely, a person might perform an action which is right in itself but he or she might have a very bad intention in so doing and might be motivated by great selfishness. Consequently, McCormick concludes: 'One's action can, therefore, be morally good, but still be morally wrong. It can be morally right, but morally bad.' He maintains that it is essential to keep this disinction in mind since 'the discussion about abortion concerns moral rightness and wrongness'. (p.180) In other words, it is not a discussion about intentions or motivation; it is about the rightness or wrongness of the action of abortion itself. Honouring this distinction, he suggests, removes a major obstacle from the conversation about abortion:

> '. . . it allows one to disagree agreeably — that is, without implying, suggesting, or predicating moral evil of the person one believes to be morally wrong. This would be a precious gain in a discussion that often witnesses this particular and serious collapse of courtesy.' (p.180)

(5) *Try to identify the core issue at stake.* McCormick is quite clear in his own mind as to what is the core issue:

> 'The core issue . . . concerns the moral claims the nascent human being . . . makes on us. Do these frequently or only very rarely yield to what appear to be extremely difficult alternatives? And above all, why or why not? That is, in my judgment, the heart of the abortion debate. It must be met head on. It is illu-

mined neither by flat statements about the inviolable rights of foetuses nor by assertions about a woman's freedom of choice. These promulgate a conclusion. They do not share with us how one arrived at it.' (pp.180-181)

(6) *Admit doubts, difficulties, and weaknesses in one's own position.*

(7) *Distinguish the formulation and the substance of a moral conviction.* McCormick explains what he means: '. . . ethical formulations, being the product of human language, philosophy, and imperfection, are only more or less adequate to the substance of our moral convictions at a given time. Ethical formulations will always show the imprint of human handling.' (p.183) However, he also adds a *caveat:*

> 'If there is a distinction between substance and formulation, there is also an extremely close — indeed inseparable — connection. One might say they are related as are body and soul. The connection is so intimate that it is difficult to know just what the substance is amid the variation of formulation. The formulation can easily betray the substance. Furthermore, because of this close connection, it is frequently difficult to know just what is changeable, what permanent. . . (To) conduct discussion as if substance and formulation were identical is to get enslaved in formulations. Such captivity forecloses conversations.' (p.184)

(8) *Distinguish morality and public policy.*

(9) *Distinguish morality and pastoral care or practice.* He gives a particularly helpful explanation of this distinction:

> 'A moral statement is . . . an abstract statement, not in the sense that it has nothing to do with real life, or with particular decisions, but in the sense that it abstracts or prescinds from the ability of this or that person to understand it and live it.
>
> Pastoral care (and pastoral statements), by contrast, looks to the art of the possible. It deals with an individual where that person is in terms of his or her strengths, perceptions, biography, circumstances (financial, medical, educational, familial, psychological). Although pastoral care attempts to expand perspectives and maximize strengths, it recognizes at times the limits of these attempts.' (p.186)

(10) *Incorporate the woman's perspective, or women's perspectives.* That many Christians would not take this for granted is evident from the fact that McCormick obviously feels a need to justify his inclusion of this rule for conversation on abortion. His 'chief reason' for including this rule is:

'Women rightly . . . insist that they are the ones who carry pregnancies and sometimes feel all but compelled to have abortions. Thus they argue two things: (1) They ought to have an influential voice in this discussion. (2) Up to and including the present, they feel they have not had such a voice.' (p.187)

Chapter 5 of this book is an indication that I am of like mind with McCormick on this matter.

McCormick's ten 'rules for conversation' are well complemented by five 'guide-lines' given by Daniel Callahan at the end of a book which is itself an excellent example of genuine dialogue in progress:

'1. There must be a more extensive discussion among those who represent the middle range of the spectrum on abortion. Although they can have some profound differences, they are normally more sympathetic toward the positions of their opposites than those who argue at the extremes. That sympathy enables them to serve as helpful rather than as hostile critics.

2. Each side should argue against the best and strongest positions of the other side, and each should also help the other to formulate the best way of putting its case. A standard tactic in many abortion polemics is to seize on the worst manifestations of behavior and logic of the opposed position and then to treat those examples as representative of the whole. Yet the most gross offenses are committed by fringe representatives, for whom the more moderate adherents in the center bear no responsibility. At the same time, it is important that those who behave badly be resolutely disavowed. It is not sufficient to condemn them and yet kindly to 'understand' them on the grounds of their sincere convictions and strong feelings.

3. Each side should reject a quest for total victory. Some degree of compromise will be necessary, not only because neither side is likely ever to command sufficient public opinion to win, but also because a due respect for the beliefs of others (even if considered wrong) is a necessary part of life in a pluralistic society.

4. Instead of beginning with those points of conviction that are the most different, discussion would best begin with those points where there is the most agreement. It is all too easy for the public, primarily exposed to black-and-white differences through the media and legislative struggles, to fail to note those areas where some degree of consensus does exist. They need to be stressed and, where possible, made the point of departure. The hardest, most divisive issues should come last, not first.

5. Each side should recognise that at least some elements of the position of the other side represent long-standing . . . values. Neither side has a monopoly either on old tradition or on the most recent new values. A synthesis of the old and the new is needed for the future, one yet to be discovered. A pro-life position does not necessarily entail a defense of the patriarchal family, a suppression of

women, or a higher defense budget. Nor does a pro-choice position on abortion necessarily entail an acceptance of infanticide, a socialist society, or a nihilistic morality. Many different combinations of values are possible and require further exploration. Nothing is more important for the quality of the debate than a rejection of the mutual stereotypes that the two sides have held about each other. The fact that they accurately reflect important regiments of the opposing sides ought not to be allowed to overshadow the larger truth that a more complex and subtle debate is emerging, one that has the possibility of breaking a now rigid and sterile mold.' (Sidney and Daniel Callahan, 1984, pp.322-323)

With reference specifically to inter-church dialogue about abortion, I would like to suggest one further 'rule for conversation':

When there is substantial disagreement between the Christian churches or between large numbers of committed and good-living Christians, this should make each church or each group of Christians hesitate to claim any more authority for their position than that it is a (not the) Christian view of the issue.

A hint of this might be found in the Council of Trent's handling of the issue of the indissolubility of marriage. Canon 7 of Session XXIV was directed against the position of Luther who held that the Church was in error in teaching that marriage came within her jurisdiction. At first reading this canon seems to be a total condemnation of remarriage after divorce. However, the Council Fathers felt they could not issue such a blanket condemnation because the Eastern Church had a limited practice of remarriage after divorce and claimed the support of St Ambrose (in fact, Ambrosiaster) and some of the other Greek Fathers for this practice. Consequently, Canon 7 was deliberately worded in such a way that it did not condemn this practice of the Eastern Church.

In our society and in our world today crimes against the human person abound in every shape and form. Those for whom the 'dignity of the human person' is a basic tenet of their belief in God need to be united. As long as we disagree in our interpretation of the implications of respect for the human person, we need to maintain a healthy element of self-criticism about our own position. None of us have a monopoly on God's Spirit. Those who differ from us also have the Spirit of God in their hearts and minds. In the 'crusade' to liberate our world from everything which violates human dignity and which oppresses the human person, we must make sure that we do not get turned aside from this common task by engaging in a kind of 'civil war'.

8

Drafting the agenda

Questions raised directly by IVF

In the course of this book we have been looking at what I have called the 'official' positions of various Christian churches dealing with IVF.

We have found that they all agree as to what must be seen as the foundational argument in favour of IVF. Since procreation is one of the 'goods' of marriage, an infertile couple have a basic right to remedy what could be termed their 'pathological' state by any means which is not detrimental to their marriage relationship nor seriously harmful to the hoped-for child or to other people. Because all the churches place such weight on procreation as one of the basic goods of marriage, this argument carries great force with them. In fact, for all but those representing the Roman Catholic position this argument is completely convincing and the churches are willing to accept IVF in principle. The 'majority' position of the Catholic Bishops' Joint Committee argues against IVF on the grounds that the separation of procreation from intercourse is bound, of its very nature, to erode married and parental love and is therefore 'unwisdom' (cf. Roman Catholic Bishops' Joint Committee, n.27). An anxiety is voiced by some members of the Anglican Working Party that IVF might be going beyond the limits of what is truly 'natural' and would perhaps have a harmful effect on people's appreciation of marriage and parenthood (cf. *Personal Origins*, n.105). It is evident that neither of these objections denies the foundational argument as such. They simply say that the conditions required by the foundational argument either *cannot* or *might* not be fulfilled.

It is clear, therefore, that any inter-church dialogue on IVF in which the Roman Catholic church is represented must include on its agenda the radical difference of view that exists between the above-mentioned Roman Catholic position and the other churches regarding the separation of procreation from intercourse. The difficulty of inter-church dialogue on this issue is heightened by two further factors: (1) the 'majority' position of the Catholic Bishops' Joint Committee does not seem to be shared by the Catholic Bishops of England and Wales; (2) because the Congregation for the Doctrine of the Faith currently plays such a major role in making sure that the Roman Catholic position is presented correctly and in its fullness, it would be difficult to imagine a local hierarchy adopting a position at variance with one of its 'official' statements, especially in view of the fact that such statements almost invariably carry some kind of stamp of papal approval.

There is a second objection raised against IVF and again it is most strongly voiced by the Roman Catholic position, even though it would seem to be shared by many Christians in the other churches as well. This objection, too, is based on a belief that seems to be shared by all the Christian churches. It is the belief that the human embryo has a God-given dignity which we are are bound to recognise. All the churches would agree, therefore, that reverence is due to the human embryo. However, the question is — what kind of reverence? Those who accept the Roman Catholic position or its equivalent would say that it is exactly the same reverence as is due to every other living human being and it is owed to the embryo from the very moment of fertilisation. Those who disagree with this would say either that it is a lesser form of reverence (and thus it would cede to the reverence due to other human beings when there is a substantial conflict of interests between them) or that the embryo is only owed full reverence at some later stage when it has developed into a human being in the full and proper sense of the word. This major divergence of view among Christians is relevant to the discussion of IVF, since IVF, as currently practised, seems to involve the production of surplus embryos which then have to be disposed of in some way or other. Therefore, some Christians who are prepared to accept IVF *in principle* might still regard its current mode of operation as unethical since it involves fertilising some ova which will subsequently be allowed to die. Moreover, the research pressures in the field of embryology raise the further ethical question as to whether these surplus embryos could be used for experimentation?

The agenda for inter-church dialogue on IVF must, therefore, also include consideration of the status of the embryo and the reverence that is due to it. Because one of the opposing views is principally represented by the Roman Catholic position, the same two complications will be present as were mentioned earlier. However, on this issue, there would seem to be much more widespread support among Roman Catholics for their church's position.

What about donor involvement? Do the churches share any common position on that issue?

They would all accept the basic principle on which the case for donor involvement is based. Where they differ is on whether the ethical acceptability of donor involvement is a conclusion which can legitimately be drawn from this principle. Most churches would either deny this or else would express serious reservations about it. The basic principle in question is really the primacy of love but in this particular context the argument in favour of donor involvement interprets it as: love is more important than genes:

> '. . . the question of genetic origin is not of fundamental moral importance, when compared with the question of how the child will be loved and cared for.'
> (*Personal Origins*, 109)

Two basic objections are raised against donor involvement and most of the churches voice either one or both of these objections: — (1) the marriage-covenant commits a couple only to have children begotten by both of them (cf. *Choices in Childlessness*, p.43); (2) children will suffer if they do not have an unimpaired sense of identity. This second objection is put most forcefully by the Roman Catholic Bishops' Joint Committee on Bio-ethical Issues: 'children have a right to be born the true child of a married couple, and thus to have an unimpaired sense of identity.' (Evidence to the Warnock Committee, n.17). Neither of these two objections rejects the basic principle itself. They both still give primacy to love. They simply argue either that the kind of love involved in the marriage-covenant rules out any form of donor-involvement or that to expose a child to the risk of having a seriously impaired sense of personal identity is not showing true love towards that child. The inter-church dialogue on IVF will need to include these two objections on its agenda.

In summary, therefore, it would seem that, if the Christian churches are to engage in dialogue about the ethical issues raised by IVF, their agenda must include three questions which are directly related to their individual approaches to this matter: —

(1) While all the churches agree that helping infertile couples remedy their condition is a good objective, what weight are they prepared to give to the claim that IVF, by separating procreation from intercourse, is bound to erode married and parental love and is therefore 'unwisdom'?

(2) While all the churches agree that reverence is owed to the embryo, are they at a complete impasse with regard to what this reverence means in practice, due to their divergent and even mutually contradictory views on the status of the embryo?

(3) While all the churches agree about the supreme importance of love in marriage, are they able to resolve their disagreement as to whether this love can be reconciled with any form of donor involvement in IVF, bearing in mind (a) the exclusive demands of the marriage covenant; and (b) the possible dangers to the IVF child's development of a healthy sense of personal identity?

Eight questions on method for the agenda

Exploring the ethical implications of IVF also raises a number of major methodological questions in the field of Christian ethics. One or two of these questions have been partially explored in this book; most have been considered too complex to be properly examined here. Among these questions, eight stand out as particularly important and will need to feature on the agenda in any future inter-church dialogue on IVF: —

(1) All the churches seem to appeal both to the nature of Christian marriage and also to the possible adverse consequences arising from either simple IVF or IVF with donor involvement. Therefore, they are combining both an essentialist and a consequentialist approach. How these two approaches relate to each other and the weight in argument to be given to each is an extremely important methodological question. Part of this discussion will need to focus on the inter-relationship between action and intention. How far does the way we behave actually shape what we are and our intentions? Do our actions merely 're-veal' or 'conceal' our true selves (depending on whether our external behaviour conforms to our internal disposition); or are our actions sometimes the very 'raw material' from which our real selves are fashioned? Initially there might be quite substantial disagreement between and even within the Christian churches on such questions as these.

(2) Even granted fairly substantial agreement on the immorality of a particular procedure in reproductive technology, some of the churches might still differ as to the practical implications of this. Some would interpret a judgement regarding the immorality of a specific practice as meaning that it can never be done; others would understand such a judgement as a statement about some of the basic values to be safeguarded but could envisage that other more fundamental values might take precedence in a particular instance. The methodological question, therefore, concerns the absoluteness of moral principles.

(3) Once again granting agreement on a particular matter on the part of those representing the various Christian churches, there is still a question as to how far the individual members of those churches believe that their consciences should be affected by the teaching of their official church representatives. This, therefore, raises the methodological question regarding the relationship between conscience and authority in matters of morality. This question is presented in its starkest form within the Roman Catholic church as is evident from the current dispute over the issue of practical and public dissent from non-infallible authoritative church teaching.

(4) Some of the working party which produced *Choices in Childlessness* voiced their conviction that 'there is a *specifically Christian* objection to the practice of AID' (italics mine). This raises the difficult methodological question as to what is specific about Christian morality. Is there a specifically Christian answer to particular issues of morality?

(5) The previous question leads naturally on to another key methodological question which would need to be faced in inter-church dialogue — the role of the Bible in helping the churches and individual Christians to make a judgement on particular moral questions. In fact, this very question caused internal division within the Methodist church when in 1980 an attempt was made to formulate a Statement putting forward a Christian understanding of sexuality that would be acceptable to all church members. As a result of this difference of opinion the Methodist Division of Social Responsibility in their revised 1982 Statement produced a most helpful comment on the use of the Bible in ethical decision-making:

'. . . the mind and will of God for the problems of today cannot be found by simply reading off doctrines and rules from Scriptural passages which appear to bear on the subject in hand . . . Christians today have to determine, by the use of the best aids available, the underlying message that the writers are conveying to those whom they are addressing, and to distinguish this from the thought-forms and language in which it is clothed . . . In the case of the Old Testament writers, they have to consider how far their message is confirmed, developed, modified or even cancelled by the teaching of the New Testament. In the case of the New Testament writers, they have to ask how far their teaching was limited by their necessarily imperfect knowledge of the world and human nature, and by the conventions and traditions of their own culture, from which they were steadily but not completely breaking free; to what extent the expectation of a speedy Second Coming formed their thought and above all how far their doctrinal teaching and their ethical counsel express a true understanding of Jesus Christ. The Biblical writers are the Church's primary and first hand witnesses to the truth as it is in Christ, and their testimony is to be both highly regarded and closely scritinized . . .' (nn.7-8)

(6) How does our theology of the Christian church and ecumenism relate the above questions, especially numbers (3), (4) and (5)? Does it imply that as long as there is serious disagreement among the churches on any moral issue of importance, no church has the right to put forward its position as '*the* Christian position' on the matter? Is 'listening' to each other's views on issues of morality not just a matter of ecumenical courtesy but a serious obligation binding on all the churches as a consequence of our belief that the Spirit is present and active among all Christians and within all Christian churches?

(7) As an extension of the above, since we believe that God's Spirit is working in the minds and hearts of all men and women of good will, does our search for a deeper understanding of God's will for humankind also seriously oblige Christian churches to adopt a similar 'listening' attitude towards what non-Christian faiths and even men and women of no religious faith have to say on the pressing moral issues facing our world today. What does this mean for inter-church dialogue on ethical issues?

(8) There are different views on specific moral questions between the Christian churches and among Christians in general. To what extent is diversity on moral issues to be welcomed as an enriching variety of complementary interpretations; to what extent is such pluralism, whether viewed as good or bad, simply inevitable as part of the ongoing process of searching for a deeper understanding of ourselves and our world; and to what extent is moral pluralism equivalent to a kind of moral relativism which would see no place for certainty about moral values or about right and wrong? How far pluralism in moral matters is acceptable clearly deserves an important place on the agenda.

The agenda and the feminist perspective

As already noted, the feminist perspective is not given its true place in the dialogue simply by including on the agenda an item entitled 'women's issues'. The feminist perspective will only be properly represented by the full involvement of women whose awareness of their special perspective as women is very much to the fore in their consciousness. Ecumenical dialogue on ethical issues will be very impoverished if women do not contribute to the full by their active speaking and listening within the dialogal process.

What about the agenda itself? Does the feminist perspective as presented in Chapter 5 raise any specific questions for ecumenical dialogue on ethical isses? Three immediately spring to mind. They all arise from general questions which were applied to the specific problem of IVF in Chapter 5:

(1) Will IVF (along with the thinking, procedures and policies linked to it) help women to become liberated from any oppression they may currently be experiencing or will it merely consolidate that oppression still further?

(2) Will it enable women to be more truly themselves as women?

(3) How does it affect our interconnectedness with each other? Does it strengthen the web of relationships or does it weaken that web and work in the direction of individualism?

The first two of these questions are drawn from the 'oppressive' side of women's experience. The third comes from the more uniquely feminist perspective. This third question might even move the dialogue on to considering such issues as (a) the way 'power' and 'competition' are operative in society; and (b) how far society can be constructed as a network of caring relationships while still respecting the individual's freedom of choice.

The feminist perspective raises three further questions for the agenda:

(1) How Christian is the institution of the family as it currently exists? Does it help individuals to become free and responsible members of the human family or is it oppressive in its over-protectiveness, shielding its members from more general social concerns?

(2) How far do the churches (perhaps only implicitly) subscribe to the view that a woman needs to be a mother if she is to be truly a woman in the full sense of the word?

(3) Are the churches willing to accept that a deliberately infertile marriage could be a true Christian marriage and a special kind of vocation in life?

9

Conclusion

Reverence for life is an attitude of wonder before the ultimate mystery of life. The whole process of the beginning of life culminating in the birth of a child is one of those privileged occasions when human consciousness feels it is in the presence of this mystery. As I conclude this book, I cannot help thinking that IVF poses a fundamental question to the Christian churches: does the intrusion of scientific technology and research into the reproductive process destroy this sense of wonder or can it provoke wonder in a new way? Putting the question even more sharply: do science and technology cause reverence to be eroded in the human heart or can they actually provide the opportunity for an entirely new human experience of reverence?

If reverence is a reaction to a human experience of depth, perhaps the churches and all of us not directly involved with IVF need to listen to what the practitioners and the couples involved are saying. They are partners in a totally new human experience. That experience might be provoking wonder and reverence in a new way. The role of the Christian churches might be to help those involved to articulate and celebrate this new experience of reverence and to share its impact and benefits with the rest of the human family. It is too early in the dialogue to say whether this is the case but at this stage it should not be excluded as a possibility.

If the Christian churches claim some expertise in the field of 'reverence', they have to face some challenging questions on this point. For instance, does reverence demand an attitude of non-interference with the basic natural processes of life and love — 'Come no nearer. Take off your shoes, for the place on which you stand is holy ground.' (Ex 3,5)? Or does reverence also embrace a practical attitude of bringing relief to couples by employing scientific technology to help them have children when their natural reproductive faculties are found to be defective — 'Is it against the law on the sabbath to do good, or to do evil; to save life, or to destroy it?' (Lk 6,9)? Or can reverence even take the form of believing that God has empowered humankind to work 'even greater wonders' (cf. Jn 14,12) than are found in creation itself. In other words, does reverence allow, and perhaps even require, humankind to alter and improve on the natural processes of reproduction, if this is considered to be humanly beneficial?

These are difficult questions. Probably all three interpretations of the demands of reverence would be able to muster some kind of Christian support. Yet Christians are also aware that each of these three forms of reverence can easily become corrupted and produce its own specific form of irreverence. For instance, the 'come no nearer' approach to reverence can easily deteriorate into the 'lack of faith' attitude of the servant who buried his talent (cf. Matt 25,14-30). The 'healing' form of reverence is in danger of following the path of Simon Magus who sought the life-giving powers of the Spirit for profitable exploitation (cf. Acts 8,9-24). And the 'even greater wonders' form of reverence can quickly fall into the trap of the rich man who wanted bigger and bigger barns for his grain (cf. Luke 12, 16-21).

As well as offering a Christian contribution to the human task of ethical analysis of the issues raised by reproductive medicine, the Christian churches should also be able to contribute from their experience of human sinfulness and divine forgiveness. Having refined what they have to offer in the purifying fire of genuine ecumenical and inter-church dialogue, they should be able to contribute a Christian view-point which is positive in its encouragement of human endeavour and yet critical of humankind's proclivity to use even the greatest discoveries of human science for purposes which are ultimately harmful.

Postscript

The Tablet (9/8/86, pp.827-828) has reported that the Congregation for the Doctrine of the Faith is putting 'the finishing touches' to a document on bioethics. Naturally, the Congregation is very anxious that bioethical issues should be considered in the light of the Christian understanding of life and death. I would wonder, however, whether the best way to achieve that aim is to issue a document on bioethics. An alternative way for the Congregation to pursue its aim would be to work in conjunction with the Secretariat for Christian Unity and explore with the other Christian churches the possibility of making an ecumenical contribution to the dialogue on bioethics. As is clear from the whole thrust of this book, I believe that the chuches themselves would benefit from the ecumenical dialogue that would be involved in preparing such a contribution. I also believe that the resulting contribution would be so much the more valuable for being able to draw on the riches of all the churches. It would be that much more Christian too!

I would even wonder whether there might not be a lesson to be learned from the Pope's invitation to representatives from all the religious faiths to join him in Assisi to pray for peace. Perhaps the day might not be too far off when a similar invitation could be issued to an inter-faith gathering to explore together where humankind is going in the whole field of bioethics. These are issues which concern the whole human family. They are of sufficient importance to call the family together to consider them.

Bibliography

WARNOCK REPORT — Department of Health and Social Security, *Report of the Committee of Inquiry into Human Fertilisation and Embryology,* Chaired by Dame Mary Warnock (HMSO, 1984)

Church reports related to IVF, abortion and ethical dialogue

BAPTIST UNION OF GREAT BRITAIN AND IRELAND

Submission to the Warnock Committee prepared by a working party under the auspices of the Baptist Union Department of Mission, and approved by the Baptist Union Council (March 1983) — unpublished
Response to the Warnock Report on behalf of The Baptist Union of Great Britian and Ireland — unpublished

BRITISH COUNCIL OF CHURCHES

Public Statements on Moral Issues, A Report from the Liaison Committee of the British Council of Churches and the Roman Catholic Church in England and Wales (Catholic Information Services, 1978)

CHURCH OF ENGLAND

Abortion: a great moral evil, Statement of Board for Social Responsibility in light of the joint statement of Catholic Archbishops of Great Britain issued on 24 January 1980
Abortion: An ethical discussion, (CIO Publishing, 1965)
General Synod: Evidence to the DHSS (Warnock) Inquiry into Human Fertilisation and Embryology. Report by the Board for Social Responsibility (March 1983)
Human Fertilisation and Embryology, The Response of the Board for Social Responsibility of the General Synod of the Church of England to the DHSS Report of the Committee of Inquiry (1984)
Personal Origins, The Report of a Working Party on Human Fertilisation and Embryology of the Board for Social Responsibility (CIO Publishing, 1985)

CHURCH OF SCOTLAND

Board of Social Responsibility: Study Group on Abortion and Report on Warnock Report, in *Reports to the General Assembly,* 1985, pp.283-291
Deliverance to General Assembly, quoted in *Life and Work,* July 1986, p.9.

CHURCH IN WALES

Advisory Commission on Church and Society: *A Contribution to the Debate on Abortion and Christian Responsibility* (September 1977) — unpublished
Human Fertilisation and Embryology, The Response of the Bench of Bishops of the Church in Wales to the Warnock Report (January 1985) — unpublished

FREE CHURCH FEDERAL COUNCIL AND THE BRITISH COUNCIL OF CHURCHES
Choices in Childlessness (1982) — The Report of a Working Party set up in July 1979 under the auspices of The Free Church Federal Council and The British Council of Churches

METHODIST CHURCH
John Atkinson (Editor), *Abortion reconsidered: The Methodist statement and its background* (Methodist Publishing House, 1977)
A Christian understanding of human sexuality, revised statement presented to the Methodist Conference in June 1982, (Methodist Publishing House, 1982)
Division of Social Responsibility, Submission to the Warnock Committee (February 1983) — unpublished
Division of Social Responsibility, Response to the Warnock Report (December 1984) — unpublished

ROMAN CATHOLIC CHURCH
Pope Paul VI, *Humanae Vitae*, (CTS, London, 1968)
'Gaudium et Spes', from *Documents of Vatican II*, ed. Abbott, (Chapman, London, 1966), pp.199-308.
Sacred Congregation for the Doctrine of the Faith, *Declaration on Procured Abortion* (1974) — English text in *Abortion and Law* (Doctrine and Life Special, Dominican Publications, Dublin, 1983)
Abortion and the Right to Live, A Joint Statement of the Catholic Archbishops of Great Britain (Catholic Information Services, 1980)
The Catholic Bishops' Joint Committee on Bio-Ethical Issues on behalf of the Catholic Bishops of Great Britain, *In Vitro Fertilisation: Morality and Public Policy*, Evidence submitted to the Warnock Committee (Catholic Information Services, 1983)
The Catholic Bishops' Joint Committee on Bio-Ethical Issues, *Response to the Warnock Report* (Catholic Information Services, 1984)
Social Welfare Commission of the Catholic Bishops' Conference (England and Wales), *Human Fertilisation: Choices for the Future* — Evidence to the Warnock Committee (Catholic Information Services, 1983)
The Joint Ethico-Medical Committee of the Catholic Union of Great Britian and the Guild of Catholic Doctors, *Submission to the Government Enquiry into Human Fertilisation and Embryology*, in Briefing, 5 August 1983 (Catholic Information Services)
The National Board of Catholic Women, *Submission to the Warnock Committee in Briefing*, 24 June 1983, (Catholic Information Services)
Statement by the Irish Bishops' Doctrinal Commission, text in *Universe*, 28 February 1986

WORLD COUNCIL OF CHURCHES
Manipulating Life: Ethical issues in genetic engineering (WCC, 1982)

Books and articles

ALBURY, Rebecca, 'Who owns the embryo?' in ARDITTI Rita, KLEIN Renate Duelli and MINDEN, Shelley (Editors), *Test-Tube Women: What Future for Motherhood?*, (Pandora Press, London, 1984) pp.54-67

ARDITTI Rita, KLEIN Renate Duelli and MINDEN, Shelley (Editors), *Test-Tube Women: What Future for Motherhood?*, (Pandora Press, London, 1984)

BATCHELOR, Edward Jr. (Editor), *Abortion: The Moral Issues* (The Pilgrim Press, New York, 1982)

BOYD, Kenneth, CALLAGHAN, Brendan, and SHOTTER, Edward, *Life Before Birth: Consensus in Medical Ethics* (SPCK, London, 1986)

BRADFORD, John, 'Development in Human Fertilisation and Embryology: Some Theological Perspectives', in *Religion and Medicine*, 1985, April, pp.16-39

CAHILL, Lisa Sowle, 'Abortion, Autonomy and Community', in CALLAHAN, Sidney and CALLAHAN, Daniel (Editors), *Abortion: Understanding Differences*, (The Hasting Center Series in Ethics, Plenum Press, New York & London, 1984) pp.261-276

CAHILL, Lisa Sowle, 'Notes in Moral Theology', in *Theological Studies*, 1985, pp.64-80

CAHILL, Lisa Sowle, 'Abortion', in MACQUARRIE, John and CHILDRESS, James (Editors), *A New Dictionary of Christian Ethics* (SCM, London, 1986), pp.1-5

CALLAHAN, Daniel, *Abortion: Law, Choice and Morality* (Collier-Macmillan, London, 1970)

CALLAHAN, Sidney and CALLAHAN, Daniel (Editors), *Abortion: Understanding Differences*, (The Hasting Center Series in Ethics, Plenum Press, New York & London, 1984)

CALLAHAN, Daniel, 'Abortion: thinking and experiencing', in *Christianity and Crisis*, Vol 32, No 23 (8/1/73) pp.295-298

CONGAR, Yves, KÜNG, Hans and O'HANLON, Daniel, *Council Speeches of Vatican II*, (Sheed & Ward, London, 1964)

CONNERY, John, *Abortion: The Development of the Roman Catholic Perspective* (Loyola University Press, Chicago, 1977)

COREA, Genoveffa, 'Egg snatchers', in ARDITTI Rita, KLEIN Renate Duelli and MINDEN, Shelley (Editors), *Test-Tube Women: What Future for Motherhood?*, (Pandora Press, London, 1984) pp.37-51

COREA Gena and others, *Man-Made Women: How new reproductive technologies affect women,* (Explorations in Feminism, Hutchinson, London, 1985)

COREA, Gena, 'The reproductive brothel', in COREA Gena and others, *Man-Made Women: How new reproductive technologies affect women,* (Explorations in Feminism, Hutchinson, London, 1985) pp.38-51

COSGRAVE, William, 'Recent Moral Thinking on Human Genetic Engineering', in *Doctrine and Life*, 1985, pp.441-449

CURRAN, Charles, 'In Vitro Fertilisation and Embryo Transfer', in *Moral Theology: A Continuing Journey* (University of Notre Dame Press, London, 1982) pp.112-140

DANIEL, William, *The Morality of In Vitro Fertilisation*, in KENNEDY, Terence (Editor), *Moral Studies: Science — Humanity — God*, (Spectrum Publications, Melbourne, 1984) pp.47-71

DUNSTAN, Gordon, 'The moral status of the human embryo: a tradition recalled', in *Journal of Medical Ethics*, 1984, pp.38-44

DUNSTAN, Gordon, 'Warnock Reviewed', in *Crucible*, 1984, pp.148-153

DUNSTAN, Gordon, 'In Vitro Fertilisation: the ethics', in *Human Reproduction*, 1986, pp.41-44

DYSON, Anthony, 'After Warnock: Questions to the Church', in *Crucible*, 1984, pp.154-161

ELSHTAIN, Jean Bethke, 'Reflections on Abortion, Values and the Family', in CALLAHAN, Sidney and CALLAHAN, Daniel (Editors), *Abortion: Understanding Differences*, (The Hasting Center Series in Ethics, Plenum Press, New York & London, 1984) pp.47-72

EVANS, Ruth, 'Ecumenical Approach to Abortion', in *The Ecumenist*, 1983, May-June, pp.64-67

EVANS, Ruth, 'From Biotechnology to Bioethics: The Shock of the Future', in *Pro Mundi Vita*, Bulletin 101, 1985/2

FLETCHER, John C., 'Reproductive Technologies' in MACQUARRIE, John and CHILDRESS, James (Editors), *A New Dictionary of Christian Ethics* (SCM, London, 1986), pp.535-539

FUCHS, Joseph, *Human Values and Christian Morality* (Gill and Macmillan, Dublin, 1970)

FUCHS, Joseph, 'Nature and Culture in Bioethics' in *Christian Ethics in a Secular Arena* (Gill and Macmillan, Dublin, 1984) pp.91-99

FUCHS, Joseph, 'Control over human life? Bioethical questions today', in *Theology Digest*, 1985, Fall, pp.247-252

GILLIGAN, Carol, *In a Different Voice; Psychological Theory and Women's Development*, (Harvard University Press, Cambridge, Massachusetts & London, England, 1982)

GUSTAFSON, James, 'A Protestant Ethical Approach' in John T Noonan (edit) *The Morality of Abortion*, (Cambridge, Mass: Harvard Univ Press, 1970) pp.101-122

HAIRE, J L M, and BOYD, J R, *Looking at Warnock — review of Response by Churches in Ireland*, private paper to Glenstal Ecumenical Conference, 1985

HARDING, Sandra, 'Beneath the Surface of the Abortion Dispute: Are Women Fully Human?' and 'Commentary on Chapter 3', in CALLAHAN, Sidney and CALLAHAN, Daniel (Editors), *Abortion: Understanding Differences*, (The Hasting Center Series in Ethics, Plenum Press, New York & London, 1984) pp.203-224, 73-80

HARING, Bernard, 'Specific Problems of Manipulation in Bioethics', in *Manipulation* (St Paul, Slough, 1975) pp.192-201

HARRIS, Peter and others, *On Human Life: An Examination of 'Humanae Vitae'*, (Burns and Oates, London, 1968)

HAUERWAS, Stanley, 'Abortion and Normative Ethics', in *Cross Currents*, 1971, Fall, pp.399-414

HAUERWAS, Stanley, 'Why Abortion is a Religious Issue', and 'Abortion: Why the Arguments Fail', in *A Community of Character: Toward a Constructive Christian Social Ethic* (University of Notre Dame Press, London, 1981) pp.196-229

HOLMES, Helen B and HOSKINS, Betty B., 'Prenatal and preconception sex choice technologies: a path to femicide?', in COREA Gena and others, *Man-Made Women: How new reproductive technologies affect women*, (Explorations in Feminism, Hutchinson, London, 1985) pp.15-29

HONEY, Colin, 'The Ethics of In Vitro Fertilisation and Embryo Transfer', in *Modern Churchman*, 1984 (2) pp.3-12

HORGAN, John (Editor), *'Humanae Vitae' and the Bishops* (Irish University Press, 1972)

Human Procreation: Ethical Aspects of the New Techniques, Report of a Working Party, Council for Science and Society (Oxford University Press, 1984)

HUME, Cardinal Basil, 'Why Warnock is wrong', in *The Times* (London), 6/6/85

IGLESIAS, Teresa, 'In Vitro Fertilisation: the major issues', in *Journal of Medical Ethics,* 1984, pp.32-37

INCE, Susan, 'Inside the surrogate industry', in ARDITTI Rita, KLEIN Renate Duelli and MINDEN, Shelley (Editors), *Test-Tube Women: What Future for Motherhood?,* (Pandora Press, London, 1984) pp.99-116

JANSSENS, L., 'Artificial Insemination: Ethical Considerations', in *Louvain Studies,* 1980, pp.3-29

JONES, D. Gareth, *Genetic Engineering* (Grove Booklets, no.25, Notts, 1978)

KIRKY, M.D., 'Bioethics of IVF — the state of the debate', in *Journal of Medical Ethics,* 1984, pp.45-48

KISHWAR, Madhu, 'The continuing deficit of women in India and the impact of amniocentesis', in COREA Gena and others, *Man-Made Women: How new reproductive technologies affect women,* (Explorations in Feminism, Hutchinson, London, 1985) pp.30-37

KLEIN, Renate Duelli, 'What's "new" about the "new" reproductive technologies?', in COREA Gena and others, *Man-Made Women: How new reproductive technologies affect women,* (Explorations in Feminism, Hutchinson, London, 1985) pp.64-73

LOCKWOOD, Michael (Editor), *Moral Dilemmas in Modern Medicine* (Oxford University Press, 1985)

LOTSTRA, Hans, *Abortion: The Catholic Debate in America* (Irvington, New York, 1985)

LUKER, Kristin, *Abortion and the Politics of Motherhood,* (University of California Press, Berkeley, Los Angeles, London, 1984)

McCORMICK, Richard, *How Brave a New World?* (SCM, London, 1981)

McCORMICK, Richard, 'Bioethics and method: Where do we start?', in *Theology Digest,* 1981, Winter, pp.303-318

McCORMICK, Richard, 'Genetic Technology and Our Common Future', in *America,* 27/4/85, pp.337-342

McCORMICK, Richard, 'Therapy or Tampering? The Ethics of Reproductive Technology', in *America,* 7/12/85, pp.396-403

McCORMICK, Richard, 'The Search for Truth in the Catholic Context', in *America*, 8/11/86, pp.276-281

McCORMICK, Richard, 'Notes in Moral Theology', in *Theological Studies*, 1975, pp.123-128; 1979, pp.99-112, 1983, p.122

MAGUIRE, Daniel C, 'The Feminisation of God and Ethics', in *Christianity and Crisis*, 15/3/82, pp.59-67

MAHONEY, John, *Bioethics and Belief* (Sheed and Ward, London, 1984)

MAHONEY, John, 'Ethical horizons of human biological development', in *The Month*, 1978, Oct, pp.329-333

MAHONEY, John, 'Warnock: A Catholic Comment', in *The Month*, 1984, Sept, pp.285-291

MAHOWALD, Mary B., 'Abortion and Equality' and 'Commentary on Chapter 4', in CALLAHAN, Sidney and CALLAHAN, Daniel (Editors), *Abortion: Understanding Differences*, (The Hasting Center Series in Ethics, Plenum Press, New York & London, 1984) pp.177-196, 109-115

MALHERBE, Jean-Francois, 'L'embryon est-il une personne?', in *Lumière et Vie*, 1985, n.172, pp.19-31

MITCHELL, Basil, 'Review-Article: Warnock', in *Modern Churchman*, 1985, pp.43-49

MONTEFIORE, Hugh, 'Experiments on Human Embryos', in *Religion and Medicine*, 1985, April, pp.2-4

MURPHY, Julie, 'Egg Farming and Women's Future', in ARDITTI Rita, KLEIN Renate Duelli and MINDEN, Shelley (Editors), *Test-Tube Women: What Future for Motherhood?*, (Pandora Press, London, 1984) pp.68-75

MURPHY, Timothy F, 'The moral significance of spontaneous abortion', in *Journal of Medical Ethics*, 1985, pp,79-83

NICHOLS, Alan, and HOGAN, Trevor, (Editors) *Making Babies: The Test Tube and Christian Ethics* (Acorn Press, Canberra, 1984 — published at the request of the Anglican Social Responsibilities Commission, Australia)

O'CONNOR, June, 'The Debate Continues: Recent Works on Abortion', in *Religious Studies Review*, 1985, April, pp.105-114

O'DONOVAN, Oliver, *Begotten or Made?* (Clarendon Press, Oxford, 1984)

O'MAHONY, Patrick and POTTS Malcolm, 'Abortion and the Soul', in *The Month*, 1967, July-Aug, pp.45-50

O'MAHONY, Patrick, 'Beginning and end of human life', in *The Month*, 1978, Nov, pp.378-382

OOMS, Theodora, 'A Family Perspective on Abortion', in CALLAHAN, Sidney and CALLAHAN, Daniel (Editors), *Abortion: Understanding Differences*, (The Hasting Center Series in Ethics, Plenum Press, New York & London, 1984) pp.81-107

PETCHESKY, Rosalind Pollack, 'Reproductive Freedom: Beyond "A Woman's Right to Choose"', in *Sign: Journal of Women in Culture and Society*, 1980, pp.661-685

PHIPPS, Terence, *Test-Tube Babies* (Catholic Truth Society, 1985)

POLLOCK, Scarlett, 'Refusing to take women seriously: "side effects" and the politics of contraception', in ARDITTI Rita, KLEIN Renate Duelli and MINDEN, Shelley (Editors), *Test-Tube Women: What Future for Motherhood?*, (Pandora Press, London, 1984) pp.138-152

RAHNER, Karl, 'The experiment with man' and 'The problem of genetic manipulation', in *Theological Investigations,* vol IX (Darton, Longman and Todd, London, 1972) pp.205-252

RAHNER, Karl, 'On bad arguments in moral theology', in *Theological Investigations,* vol XVIII, pp.74-85

RAMSEY, Paul, *Prefabricated Man* (Yale University Press, New Haven and London, 1970)

RAMSEY, Paul, 'Abortion: A Review Article', in *Thomist,* 1973, pp.174-226

REACH, Warren T. (Editor) *Encyclopedia of Bioethics* (Collier-Macmillan, London, 1978), vol II pp.485-493, 513-578; vol IV pp.1439-1470

REIDY, Maurice, (Editor) *Ethical Issues in Reproductive Medicine* (Gill and Macmillan, Dublin, 1982)

ROGGENCAMP, Viola, 'Abortion of a special kind: male sex selection in India', in ARDITTI Rita, KLEIN Renate Duelli and MINDEN, Shelley (Editors), *Test-Tube Women: What Future for Motherhood?,* (Pandora Press, London, 1984) pp.266-277

ROTHMAN, Barbara Katz, 'The meaning of choice in reproductive technology', in ARDITTI Rita, KLEIN Renate Duelli and MINDEN, Shelley (Editors), *Test-Tube Women: What Future for Motherhood?,* (Pandora Press, London, 1984) pp.23-33

ROTHMAN, Barbara Katz, 'The products of conception: the social context of reproductive choice', in *Journal of Medical Ethics,* 1985, pp.188-193

ROWLAND, Robyn, 'Motherhood, patriarchal power, alienation and the issue of "choice" in sex preselection', in COREA Gena and others, *Man-Made Women: How new reproductive technologies affect women,* (Explorations in Feminism, Hutchinson, London, 1985) pp.74-87

SEGERS, Mary C., 'Abortion and the Culture; Towards a Feminist Perspective', in CALLAHAN, Sidney and CALLAHAN, Daniel (Editors), *Abortion: Understanding Differences,* (The Hasting Center Series in Ethics, Plenum Press, New York & London, 1984) pp.229-252

SHEA, M C, 'Embryonic life and human life', in *Journal of Medical Ethics,* 1985, pp.205-209

SINGER, P. and WELLS, D., *The Reproductive Revolution* (Oxford University Press, 1984)

SOLOMON, David, 'Philosophers on Abortion', in MANIER, E, LIU, W, and SOLOMON D, (Editors), *Abortion: New Directions for Policy Studies* (University of Notre Dame Press, Notre Dame, Indiana, 1977) pp.159-167

SPECK, Peter, 'Issues on Human Fertilisation and Embryology', in *Religion and Medicine,* 1985, April, pp.5-15

STACEY, Margaret, 'Commentary', (on Rothman 1985) in *Journal of Medical Ethics,* 1985, pp.193-195

STEINBACHER, Roberta, and HOLMES, Helen B., 'Sex choice: survival and sisterhood', in COREA Gena and others, *Man-Made Women: How new reproductive technologies affect women,* (Explorations in Feminism, Hutchinson, London, 1985) pp.52-63

TORRANCE, Thomas F., *Test-Tube Babies* (Scottish Academic Press, Edinburgh, 1984)

VARGA, Andrew C., *The Main Issues in Bioethics* (Fowler Wright, Leominster, 1980)

Acknowledgements

The publishers acknowledge with thanks permission to quote as follows:

Catholic Truth Society (S345), *Abortion and the Right to Live: a joint statement*, 1980

Central Board of Finance of the Church of England, *Abortion: an ethical discussion; Human Fertilisation and Embryology; Personal Origins*

Church of Scotland Board of Social Responsibility, *Report of Study Group on Abortion* and *on the Warnock Report*

Dominican Publications, Ireland, *Declaration on Procured Abortion,* from Austin Flannery OP (ed), *Vatican Council II: More Post Conciliar Documents*

Gill and Macmillan Ltd, Joseph Fuchs, *Human Values and Christian Morality*

Joint Bio-ethical Committee of Catholic Bishops of Great Britain, *In vitro fertilisation: morality and public policy*, 1983

Methodist Publishing House, John Atkinson (ed), *Abortion Reconsidered*, submission to the Warnock Committee; *Revised Statement*, 1982

Plenum Publishing Corporation, Sidney and Daniel Callahan, *Abortion: Understanding Differences*

SCM Press Ltd and Doubleday Inc, Richard McCormick, *How Brave a New World?*

Index